SELF-DISCLOSURE IN PSYCHOTHERAPY

Self-Disclosure in Psychotherapy

BARRY A. FARBER

THE GUILFORD PRESS
New York   London

© 2006 The Guilford Press
A Division of Guilford Publications, Inc.
72 Spring Street, New York, NY 10012
www.guilford.com

Printed in the United States of America

This book is printed on acid-free paper.

Last digit is print number: 9 8 7 6 5 4 3 2 1

Library of Congress Cataloging-in-Publication Data

Farber, Barry A. (Barry Alan), 1947–
    Self-disclosure in psychotherapy / Barry A. Farber.
      p. ; cm.
    Includes bibliographical references and index.
    ISBN-13: 978-1-59385-323-5 (alk. paper)
    ISBN-10: 1-59385-323-8 (alk. paper)
    1. Psychotherapy. 2. Self-disclosure. 3. Psychotherapist and patient.
I. Title.
    [DNLM: 1. Psychotherapy. 2. Professional–Patient Relations. 3. Self
Disclosure.   WM 420 F219s 2006]
    RC480.5.F323 2006
    616.89′14—dc22

                                            2006010618

Excerpt from "The Stranger" by Billy Joel used by permission.
Copyright © 1977 by Impulsive Music. All rights reserved.

"Losing My Religion." Words and music by William Berry, Peter Buck,
Mike Mills, and Michael Stipe. © 1991 Night Garden Music. All Rights on
Behalf of Night Garden Music. Administered by Warner-Tamerlane
Publishing Corp. All Rights Reserved. Used by Permission. PR1217-0001

For my mom.

Thanks for all the love, humor, and chocolate—
Who could ask for more?

About the Author

Barry A. Farber, PhD, received his degree in clinical psychology from Yale University. Currently, he is a Professor of Psychology and Education at Teachers College, Columbia University. He has twice served as Chair of the Counseling and Clinical Psychology Department at Teachers College, and has been the Program Coordinator and Director of Training in the Clinical Psychology Program since 1990. Dr. Farber serves on the editorial boards of several professional journals and maintains a small private practice of psychotherapy in Mamaroneck, New York. He has written three previous books, most recently the coedited volume (with Debora C. Brink and Patricia M. Raskin) *The Psychotherapy of Carl Rogers: Cases and Commentary* (published by Guilford). Dr. Farber has written articles on stress and burnout, psychological-mindedness, therapist and patient representations, career motivations of therapists, and the therapist as an attachment figure. He is currently working on a book about psychologically astute rock and roll lyrics.

Preface

Sometime in the late 1980s I was talking with some of my graduate students in the Clinical Psychology Program at Teachers College at Columbia University about learning to do psychotherapy, and about the specific difficulty of knowing when to stay silent and when to push gently for patients to say more. We began discussing what patients found hard to speak about in therapy. Some students thought "sex" would be highest on the list of avoided or difficult-to-discuss topics others thought "angry feelings about one's therapist." So Freudian, we thought: sex and aggression. And then we wondered: What do patients speak about most? Is it feeling depressed? Feeling disconnected? Anger at parents? A sense of unfulfillment in life?

After the jibes about how our guesses were great examples of our own defenses (projection) and assumptions, we agreed on two points: first, that there were likely to be some normative patterns around disclosure, but second, that what patients do and don't speak about in therapy also depends on many factors. Some of these factors, we thought, would include therapeutic orientation, length of time spent in treatment, strength of the therapeutic relationship, diagnoses or presenting problems, and demographic variables, such as patient age, gender, and ethnicity. We also imagined that the therapist's style, including his or her tendency to be self-disclosing, would have an effect on patient disclosure patterns.

Looking into it, I discovered that there was almost no published scholarly work on this topic. Despite the fact that the currency in psychotherapy essentially consists of spoken words, and despite the fact that psychotherapy research was a strongly established tradition by the late 1980s, very few studies had investigated patient disclosure in therapy. Although Sidney Jourard had done some intriguing work on interpersonal disclosure in the 1960s and 1970s, this line of inquiry hadn't been extended to the psychotherapeutic setting.

I decided to embark on a series of studies that ultimately included work on patient, therapist, and supervisory disclosure, and involved participants from as close as New York and as far away as Hawaii and Israel. Much of this work has been presented at professional conferences over the years, most often at the meetings of the Society for Psychotherapy Research. And much has been published in professional journals as well.

Why, then, a book? One reason is to integrate the work that has been done on various forms of therapy disclosure over the years. For the most part, this literature has tended to focus on disclosure patterns specific to the patient, therapist, supervisor, or supervisee. But there are commonalities among these findings—for example, the role of shame in nondisclosure—that are typically overlooked. A book allows similarities and differences among the participants in therapy and supervision to be explored in some detail. A second reason for writing a book is to bring together the findings of several research teams, most notably those of Clara Hill at the University of Maryland, College Park, Bill Stiles at Miami University in Ohio, Anita Kelly at Notre Dame University, Nick Ladany at Lehigh University, and my own at Teachers College. Each has done some important work, and it was time for all of it (or at least most of it) to be assembled and discussed within a single volume.

A third, related reason is to bring together research findings, clinical observations, and theoretical perspectives on disclosure-related issues in therapy. As is true for so many psychological phenomena—diagnosis comes to mind as an example—these viewpoints tend too often to be kept separate. Those who privilege one way of understanding certain issues too rarely bother to read about, much less appreciate, other perspectives. Thus, with rare exception, work on disclosure has tended to be compartmentalized. Clinicians writing about therapist disclosure have generally been uninformed about the empirical research on this topic; researchers have often been surprisingly unaware of the abundant theoretical literature on the very questions they are studying. In particular, too many researchers regard psychoanalytic literature as unworthy of their attention. It's also true that too many psychoanalytic theorists have apparently avoided not only researchers' contributions to the literature on disclosure but also clinical ideas and theories proffered by those from differing theoretical traditions. A book allows rich clinical traditions to be valued side by side with significant research findings.

A fourth reason for this book was that it provided an opportunity to consider the historical context for the burgeoning interest in disclosure issues in the United States. As I describe in the first chapter, disclosure has become an area of interest not just in psychotherapy but in a wide variety of media, including books, television, and the Internet. Professional presentations and articles typically don't permit the luxury of contextualizing research and theoretical findings, of locating them at a certain place in history.

Mostly, though, I felt a new book on this topic was overdue. This book is the first comprehensive look at disclosure issues in therapy since Stricker and Fisher's edited volume on this topic, *Self-Disclosure in the Therapeutic Relationship*, in 1990. A great deal has occurred since the publication of that seminal work, including the first empirical studies of supervisor and supervisee disclosure; extensive research on patient and therapist disclosure; far greater acceptance among therapists of multiple theoretical traditions of the mutative possibilities inherent in therapeutic disclosures; substantially increased clinical interest in the ways in which culture and ethnicity affect patient and therapist disclosure; influential research on the psychological and physiological benefits of written expression; and heady debates on the relative benefits of "expression versus repression" in the wake of trauma. As important and heuristically valuable as Stricker and Fisher's book was, all but one chapter focused on therapist disclosure. This proportion reflected accurately the state of the knowledge and the boundaries of clinical interest in disclosure at that time.

I've organized this book to reflect what I believe is now the state of affairs in this field. I've begun with a chapter that provides some historical context for the current interest in the topic of interpersonal disclosure. Chapter 1 traces the history of self-disclosure research within the social psychological and psychotherapeutic communities, reviews the various attempts to define the concept, surveys contemporary forms of disclosure across various media, and provides an overview of the positive and negative consequences of interpersonal disclosure. Chapter 2 focuses on patient disclosure per se (including nonverbal disclosure), with a review of the various factors that affect the probability of its occurrence (including legal issues surrounding confidentiality) and a discussion of the typical ways that patients and therapists negotiate the ambivalence that typically surrounds decisions to disclose.

Chapters 3, 4, and 5 focus on several other aspects of patient disclosure. Chapter 3 reviews the burgeoning empirical literature on this topic, with particular attention paid to what patients do and don't disclose in therapy. Chapter 4 examines the controversy over the specific effects of disclosure, namely, whether (and under what circumstances) disclosing is an effective strategy for ameliorating stress. Chapter 5 tackles the growing topic of multiculturalism—specifically, the ways in which the cultural traditions and values of Asian American, African American, and Latino communities in the United States influence patient disclosure.

The next three chapters are devoted to therapist disclosure. Chapter 6 reviews the controversial history of therapist disclosure, with an emphasis on the divergent ways that it has been thought about within the psychoanalytic community. Chapter 7 provides an overview of the research on therapist disclosure; the emphases here are on examining the most common forms of therapist disclosure and their effects on therapeutic process and outcome. Chapter 8 examines various clinical perspectives on disclosure, especially therapists' views on whether and when disclosures are helpful. This chapter also discusses how special circumstances (e.g., therapist pregnancy or illness) affect the timing and nature of certain disclosures. Chapter 9 surveys the growing literature on supervisee and supervisor disclosure. Finally, Chapter 10 attempts to highlight the major findings, trends, implications, and directions for this growing field.

I've used many clinical examples in this book. Some have been quoted (with acknowledgment) from other sources. Some case material or anecdotes were provided by colleagues or students when they became aware of this project. In these cases, I've changed significant details about the clinical participants in order to safeguard their identity and privacy. I've reviewed these changes with these colleagues and students to ensure that all possible identifying material has been deleted. Similarly, the clinical material that comes from my own practice has been significantly modified in the service of confidentiality. The poem at the end of the book, provided by a patient of mine, is used with explicit permission.

I've also used a number of quotes from books, movies, and rock songs. I'll simply say that I enjoy finding wisdom in whatever sources are available, and that those sources are not restricted to professional books and journal articles.

I struggled with the choice of using "patient" or "client" throughout this book. The voluminous psychoanalytic literature on therapist disclosure uses the word "patient." On the other hand, much of the research on patient, therapist, supervisor, and supervisee disclosure has been published in counseling journals, which prefer the word "client." I've ended up primarily using "patient," but I've also used "client" at times, and they're meant to be read as synonyms.

Writing this book has been a long but very fine journey, full of fulfilling and productive collaborations with many smart colleagues and talented graduate students.

Jesse Geller served on my dissertation committee at Yale University in 1978; he is now a valued colleague and friend. Jesse's comments on this book, like those on other pieces I've written (or those we've coauthored), have been wise, thoughtful, and reflective of his remarkable range of knowledge. Roni Tower is also a colleague at Teachers College whose support and encouragement have been invaluable; and Dinelia Rosa, Director of our student clinic, has facilitated my research over the years and provided especially helpful advice on the chapter on multicultural issues. Sandra Azar at Pennsylvania State University has made consistently excellent suggestions on many aspects of this project. I also feel indebted to those colleagues who've critiqued (in the best sense of the word) my research at professional conferences: Clara Hill at the University of Maryland, College Park, David Orlinsky at the University of Chicago, and Bill Stiles at Miami University in Ohio have been consistently gracious and helpful.

George Goldstein, former Director of the Westchester Center for the Study of Psychoanalysis and Psychotherapy and dear friend, was an astute reader of the manuscript; his comments were a great help in preparing final revisions. Likewise, Sam Menahem, President of the Association for Spirituality and lifelong friend, furthered my thinking about many of the issues in this book via many provocative and enjoyable conversations. Susan Alexander, Ghislaine Boulanger, Billie Pivnick, Jane Roth, and Saul Scheidlinger—excellent psychologists all—provided references, ideas, suggestions, and wisdom. Diana Fosha and Stephanie Fagin-Jones were kind and courageous enough to provide case examples of therapist disclosure.

I have also profited greatly from my conversations and friendship with two former students. Clarissa Bullitt, with whom I've collaborated on several articles on gender and defenses, is able to suffuse her keen understanding of psychological issues with an extraordinary degree of literary knowledge and sensitivity. Betsy Glaser is as gifted a clinician as I've ever known.

I'm very appreciative of my students who've worked with me on these issues, including those (Kathryn Berano, Joe Capobianco, Sherrie Kim, Dailey Pattee, and Alice Sohn) who in recent years have presented our work at professional conferences. Each has been a pleasure to work with and each has contributed a great deal to my thinking on these issues. Very special thanks to two students who have worked as my research assistants on this book, Jesse Metzger and Rachel Khurgin, doctoral students in the Clinical Psychology Program at Teachers College. Both write beautifully, edit carefully, read thoughtfully, and offered consistently excellent suggestions about the organization and content of this work. Sincere thanks also to Kara Graziano, who was so conscientious and appropriately obsessive about keeping my extensive number of references in order. Rebecca Shulevitz is the secretary for our Clinical Psychology Program at Teachers College. She is the best secretary any faculty member could ever hope for, but her unfailingly kind assistance to me and every other member of the program goes far beyond that title.

Kathryn Berano did a substantial amount of the background work for the chapter on multicultural issues in patient disclosure, as did Joe Capobianco for the chapter on historical perspectives on therapist disclosure. Jean Seibel, a talented dance therapist contributed significantly to the section on disclosure in nonverbal therapies. I am grateful to each. I am also very grateful to Jim Nageotte, Senior Editor at The Guilford Press. He has been a knowledgeable, generous, and patient guide throughout this process. Thanks also to Jane Keislar, editorial assistant at Guilford, for her assistance in taking me and this book through the final stages of production.

My family, as always, has been supportive and loving. They have endured my nearly constant presence at multiple computers in multiple rooms of our house, including those (my son has reminded me) that don't belong to me. So, thank you, dear April, Alissa, and David. And thank you, dear Mom. And dear Pops. To health and the love of family.

Contents

CHAPTER 1

The Nature of Self-Disclosure

No man can come to know himself except as an outcome of
disclosing himself to another person.
—JOURARD (1971b, p. 6)

When the first man opened his eyes and discovered he was naked,
he tried to conceal himself even from the sight of his maker; so
diligence in hiding was born almost when the world was born.
—ECO (1996, p. 112)

The primary aim of this book is to examine the nature of self-disclosure in
psychotherapy. More specifically, this book addresses self-disclosure from
several perspectives: that of patient to therapist, therapist to patient, supervisor to supervisee, and supervisee to supervisor.

Although there are significant differences in the structure and dynamics of each of these relationships that affect the tendency to disclose personal material—for example, the clinical space available for patients to tell
their stories and secrets should be far broader than that for therapists—all
interpersonal disclosures share common elements. All disclosures reflect
decisions about the boundaries between the private self and the outer
world. All revolve around a basic question: What elements of our private
world will we express to the outer world? Most often, disclosures involve
negotiating an appropriate balance between the helpfulness of sharing a
part of ourselves with another and the inappropriateness or even danger of
overdoing it, of perhaps sharing too much too soon. Psychotherapy, a place
of nearly total confidentiality, provides a rich and unique setting in which
to examine this quintessentially human conflict. In doing so, in studying the
nature and consequences of disclosure, we can enrich our understanding of
interpersonal relations in general and of something fundamental about the
psychotherapeutic process.

The therapist's office seems a natural arena in which to examine issues of self-disclosure. It is the place in which patients are expected and sometimes exhorted to confide their secrets, their suppressed memories, their hidden (and not-so-hidden) feelings, their vaguely remembered dreams, their most shameful fantasies, their immediate experiences. Patients in therapy come to talk about themselves, and, in fact, therapy is one of those rare situations in life where talking about oneself is not only considered appropriate but necessary.

The therapist's office is also a place in which therapists must consider what they will disclose to their patients, a topic that has attracted enormous interest and debate within the psychotherapeutic community over the past few decades. Controversy has raged over such questions as: What constitutes therapist disclosure? Is therapist disclosure helpful or ultimately and essentially narcissistic? And, if helpful, which kinds of disclosure are most useful and under what conditions?

Relatedly, though often overlooked in discussions regarding disclosure in psychotherapy, therapy supervisors and supervisees must decide what they will and will not disclose to the other. These decisions affect not only their relationship to one another but also the nature of the psychotherapeutic treatment being offered by the supervisee.

In this first chapter, I discuss the general nature of self-disclosure, including a short history of attempts to investigate it empirically. I speculate as to why self-disclosure has become more prominent in American culture in recent years, enumerate some of the positive and negative consequences of this phenomenon, and review the debate in the field over expressing versus repressing one's thoughts and feelings. This chapter, then, provides a context for subsequent chapters that examine the nature of self-disclosure in psychotherapy per se.

We feel close to some people, like family members, because we have grown up with them or simply because the role demands it. We feel close to others, including colleagues, friends, and lovers, because they have opened themselves up to us. They have told us their story. They have let us in on their world, telling us about themselves, including their feelings, thoughts, and desires. They may even have let us know of their deepest fears and their most traumatic experiences. Their self-disclosures make us feel special or privileged, and we often respond by sharing deeper parts of ourselves.

But the process, of course, is typically more complicated than this. The person disclosing to us may well be wondering, even as he or she is sharing an intimate feeling or family secret, whether it is appropriate or worth the risk; he or she may be feeling shame, guilt, or confusion or perhaps pride, love, or lust. This person may want affirmation or information or advice—or may be hoping that this sharing will lead to reciprocal sharing but also feeling apprehensive that it might not. He or she may be fearful that this private information will be shared with others. He or she may also be imagining what we as the recipient of this information are now thinking or feeling—wondering whether we really care and understand or whether we are going to be judgmental or critical. And, as the recipient of this disclosure, we may also be full of multiple overlapping thoughts and questions: Why is he or she sharing this with me? Is it appropriate? Is it truthful? Do I want to hear this? How shall I respond? Who else has he or she shared this with? Is this the start of something big?

Ask people about their experiences of disclosing to another and you get a sense of the variability and complexity of the self-disclosure process. These comments—edited and modified for the purposes of confidentiality (as are all my examples in this book)—are drawn from conversations with friends, students, patients, and supervisees:

> "I've become aware that some people are un-self-conscious about sharing horrendous, shameful events in their lives. I'm amazed at this and never sure whether they're being courageous or naive."

> "Here's my image of myself as a discloser: I offer 80% of myself almost promiscuously. I'm open, share a great deal of myself to most everyone, almost invariably give thoughtful honest answers to even moderately intimate questions. But the other 20%? Oh my. You have to fight every inch to get every percentage point after that."

> "Some of the absolute best moments of my life have been when I've shared something hard and the other person really gets it. And some of the worst moments are when I've shared something deep and the person hasn't understood the meaning of what I'm doing or the gift I'm offering."

> "About the best thing about being in a clinical psychology program is the opportunity to talk almost constantly about the most intimate things with other students, faculty, and even supervisors. It feels so good on so many levels to be real and to be close to others."

> "Sometimes I think I became a therapist just so I could hear all those great secrets."

Clearly, the meaning and value of self-disclosure varies greatly among individuals and also varies within individuals as a function of context (time, place, mood, and to whom one is disclosing). Indeed, self-disclosure is a somewhat elusive and complex concept. The *New York Times*'s retired columnist and word maven William Safire defined disclosure as "to make known what was previously unpublished, deliberately held back or kept secret" (1999, p. 47), a definition that speaks to the inevitable dialectic between what is and what is not said. Disclosure, in this sense, "undoes" silence, distance, or ignorance. It implies a distinction between what we think and what we say. In this sense, it is a phenomenon that mediates the relationship between one's inner, personal self and the outer world.

Sidney Jourard (1971b), the progenitor of contemporary research on this topic, defined self-disclosure as permitting one's true self to be known to others. This is a seemingly elegant and straightforward definition, involving some degree of intentionality, but it sidesteps the intriguing question of how to define the "true self." Writing before the dawn of postmodernism or of discussions of the nature of multiple selves (e.g., Mitchell, 1993), Jourard did not engage in philosophical discourses of this sort. What he did suggest (1971b) was that individuals need to find the courage to share deeply held thoughts and feelings with others. Implicitly, Jourard reminds us that disclosures can range from the mundane to the profound and that consistent but superficial disclosures still leave us strangers to others. He also believed that each of us is constantly confronted with an existential challenge: "Shall we permit our fellow persons to know us as we are, or shall we seek instead to remain an enigma, an uncertain quality, wishing to be seen as something we are not"? (p. iii). Here, of course, Jourard observes that silence is also a choice, a decision with its own implications, including the possibility that we would not just be "unknown" but "misknown," prey perhaps to others' assumptions or projections.

Furthermore, Jourard conceived of self-disclosure as a circular and interactive phenomenon, moving continuously between the self and another. It is only in this manner, thought Jourard, that one could honor the maxim of "know thyself," for in revealing oneself to another one necessarily learns about oneself. In disclosing, we often become aware of thoughts, feelings, and behaviors we did not know we had. And, as we further consider what we've said, new memories and thoughts come to mind. Furthermore, in revealing to another we are confronted with new information—body language or questions that lead to clarifications of what we've just conveyed. Or, the person to whom we've disclosed reveals something that stimulates more of our own thoughts and memories. Our self is constituted through interactions with others, and we move toward greater self-knowledge by understanding the nature of self in relationship to other.

The Johari window (Luft, 1969; see Figure 1.1) is a simple but compelling means of categorizing several types of secrecy and disclosure. This figure, named after its two authors (Joseph Luft and Harry Ingham), suggests that openness in relationships can be conceptualized as consisting of four windows, or quadrants:

1. *That which is known to both oneself and others (open).* When individuals first meet, this window is necessarily small but enlarges as time goes on and as personal information is shared. In intimate relationships, includ-

	Known to Self	Not Known to Self
Known to Others	Open Self	Blind Self
Not Known to Others	Hidden Self	Unknown Self

FIGURE 1.1. The Johari window.

ing marriage, friendships, and long-term therapy, this window is relatively large and, ideally, is constantly enlarging.

2. *That which is not known to others but is known to oneself (hidden).* This window represents aspects about oneself that are not shared. This window is likely to be radically different in different relationships and is likely to be smallest in intimate relationships. However, for virtually everyone, this window is never entirely closed even in the closest of relationships. That is, we all tend to keep parts of ourselves hidden.

3. *That which is not known to oneself but is known to others (blind).* This window represents aspects of oneself unknown to the self but seen by others. Examples range from the trite (e.g., having bits of food on one's face while eating) to the relatively profound (e.g., a significant degree of anxiety or discomfort in social situations; a heavy dose of defensiveness when being evaluated or supervised). Others may struggle to present this information in a tactful enough way so that it can be heard and accepted.

4. *That which is not known to oneself nor others (unknown).* In this window or quadrant is information that is unknown to self and others. Some individuals, for example, have a history of childhood sexual or physical abuse that they have no conscious memory of; they have successfully repressed this experience (although it may color their relationships with others). The existence of material within this quadrant may sometimes be inferred by one's symptoms (e.g., posttraumatic stress disorder), but the nature of such information only becomes apparent in retrospect, after it has been revealed. Discussing one's dreams with another person may also yield information about oneself that has been previously unknown to either the self or the other.

As Larson (1993) has noted, therapy can be viewed as a process of expanding the first quadrant (information available to self and others) while contracting the others. However, despite its heuristic value, the Johari window is limited in its capacity to describe the complexity of the information it attempts to categorize. First, its categorical design precludes differentiation among the various bits of information contained within each quadrant. For example, although "bad breath" and "quick-tempered" might both be accurately classified within the blind quadrant, we are unable to perceive the degree to which an individual is differentially blind to each. Second, the design assumes a degree of absoluteness that doesn't truly exist in the world. That is, the "known to self" versus "not known to self" and the "known to others" versus "not known to others" dichotomies are more realistically seen as existing on a continuum.

Finally, the assumption of discrete, mutually exclusive categories violates what most of us, especially therapists, realize: that some "truths" that are known to the self may be intertwined with truths that are not known to the self, or may preclude awareness of still other truths. Let us say that a wife leaves her husband because he cheated on her. She believes she left because of his infidelity (a known-to-self truth). But perhaps she had also unconsciously sabotaged the relationship prior to the affair, wishing to escape the marriage because she felt unfulfilled (an unknown-to-self truth). The truth of the reason she left her husband may therefore partially reside in two categories rather than one. It is a formidable task in all interpersonal situations, including therapy, to disentangle competing truths.

Attempts at categorization aside, questions about what, why, and to whom we confide have engaged both social and clinical psychologists for nearly half a century. Such questions have also engaged writers and philosophers and, indeed, most psychologically minded individuals. Wondering what we should and shouldn't tell others about ourselves, wondering about the meaning and veracity of what others tell us, and wondering about the effects of revealing our private thoughts are central concerns to most self-aware people.

WHY IS SELF-DISCLOSURE IN THERAPY
NOW A "HOT TOPIC"?

Therapists are fond of asking the question "why now?" in response to a patient's acknowledgment that he or she has finally acted a certain way (e.g., confronted a partner about a long-standing concern; decided to come to therapy after years of considering it). We might ask, then, why the issue of self-disclosure seems to be of particular interest at this time to the psychotherapeutic community. In attempting to answer this question, however, we need to keep in mind that the issue has never entirely been out of awareness—from its inception, psychotherapy has encouraged its consumers to withhold nothing from the therapist, that is, to disclose everything. "Say whatever comes to mind, without censorship" is the essence of Freud's "fundamental rule." To a great extent, psychotherapy in all its forms has always been based on a patient's willingness to disclose personal, often shameful, information.

Nevertheless, what is clear to most observers is that the field of psychotherapy has shifted dramatically in the past few decades from a primary focus upon drive-related intrapsychic issues to a primary focus upon interpersonal issues. The therapist, especially in psychodynamically oriented therapy, is no longer seen as the sole expert in the room, observing and interpreting a patient's dynamics or the nature of the transference; rather, he or she is part of a system, a two-person field, in which both participants cocreate meaning and both observe the nature of what is being created. Issues of attachment, internalization, attunement, and intersubjectivity are now essential aspects of many therapists' work. As part of this trend, the nature of communication between the two participants in therapy—what each does and does not tell the other, especially feelings and thoughts about the other and the relationship—has become a far more prominent part of the therapeutic process. Thus, contemporary therapists are not only placing more emphasis on how patients are revealing themselves in therapy but also questioning themselves about what, when, and why they should reveal to their patients.

To a certain extent, this shift in psychotherapy toward a greater emphasis on interpersonal issues and disclosure is a reflection of changes in the wider culture. In reaction to increasing feelings of anonymity or detachment resulting from the frenzied pace of technology, the perceived lack of a sense of community, and the seeming ubiquity of a shopping mall culture, individuals in our society seem to be craving more personal information about one another. In this regard, Harry Guntrip, a noted figure in the British school of object relations, began his book *Personality Structure and Human Interaction* with the following quote: "History shows that scientific effort tends to flow along channels leading to discoveries which contemporary society consciously needs and is ready to pay for" (Association of Scientific Workers, cited in Guntrip, 1961, p. 25). Guntrip's point was that following two great wars the world was primed for a system of psychology that emphasized not aggression or sexuality but rather the origins of and need for effective interpersonal relationships. Over the past few decades, clinical psychology has moved away from a focus on an impersonal "id" (the source of drives) to a focus on the ways in which we symbolize our relatedness to others.

More recently, in reaction to environmental disasters and fears of terrorism, many individuals have hungered for greater intimacy. In the wake of 9/11, many began sharing political, psychological, religious, and existential convictions in far greater depth and with a far greater number of people. A similar phenomenon was observed following the devastation wrought in 2005 by hurricanes Katrina and Rita.

But beyond the sharing that typically occurs in the aftermath of tragedies, many people in this country have seemed eager in recent years to disclose remarkably intimate and sensitive aspects of their lives, including details about such topics as abuse or addiction. Reflecting this need (or perhaps catalyzing it), confessional books, TV magazine programs (*20-20*; Barbara Walters' specials), talk shows (e.g., *Oprah*; *Dr. Phil*), reality series (*Survivor*), tabloid newspaper columns, radio call-in shows, popular magazines (*People*), and online diaries and chat rooms have all propagated a "tell-all" mentality. Even nominees for local and national elections seem to be expected to reveal far more details about their personal lives now than they were even a few decades ago. To be sure, many disclosures of this type are in the service of personal, e.g., political or social, gain rather than in the service of intimacy, but the fact remains that sharing more of ourselves with others has become more normative. As the novelist Richard Russo observed in a recent novel: "My daughter belongs to a talk show generation that seems to be losing its ability to discriminate between public and private woes" (1998, p. 216).

Arguably, some of these changes began in the 1960s. The politics and sensibilities of the 1960s—civil rights, women's rights, sexual openness, the dawning of multiculturalism—offered, and at times demanded, new ways of accepting and understanding others. Along with this focus came an emphasis on learning about and sharing more of ourselves with others. Moreover, the "others" in this equation were not restricted to family, lovers, or best friends but, in fact, extended to acquaintances as well as strangers—indeed, the universe of others. In the service of the principle that "All men are brothers," the boundaries between private and public knowledge began to collapse. The popularity of encounter groups in the late 1960s and early 1970s exemplified a tell-all philosophy, an ethos of "if you think it or feel it, say it." Another telling phrase of this era was: "Let it all hang out." Less influential but also consistent with this ethos was the burgeoning of the "confessional" poetry movement during this decade, as seen for example in the works of Robert Lowell and Sylvia Plath. Similarly, it was during this era that highly popular singer-songwriters made their mark, most notably Bob Dylan, Paul Simon, and Joni Mitchell. Although Dylan was the most explicitly political of this group, all were seen as telling intensely personal stories through their music.

It would also be possible to argue that the watershed event during the mid-20th century vis-à-vis disclosure was the publication in 1948 by Alfred Kinsey and associates of *Sexual Behavior in the Human Male* and, 5 years later, of *Sexual Behavior in the Human Female*. At the time these works came out, public morality precluded open discussion of sexuality, especially sexual practices. The publication of these books harkened the abolition of the last taboo: talking about sex and sexuality.

Freud, Kinsey, and the cataclysms of the 1960s all had effects on public consciousness, including decisions about the boundaries of public disclosure. In his book *How We Got Here: The 70s: The Decade That Brought You Modern Life (for Better or Worse)*, Frum (2000) suggested that by the 1970s most people in this country had begun to accept the idea that good mental health required "excruciating" public confessions, an idea exemplified by Betty Ford's acknowledgment of her drug and alcohol addiction and by other celebrities' similar public disclosures. According to Frum, virtually everyone in the country accepted the premise that it was dangerous to keep feelings bottled up. By the late 1990s, noted Michener (1995), the publishing world had not only embraced celebrity memoirs (unexpurgated stories about the "pain behind the fame") but had given its unreserved blessing to a flood of just-plain-folks memoirs—intensely personal accounts by non-celebrities about growing up in severely disturbed families and overcoming serious psychological trauma.

Still, as noted earlier, it would be a mistake to imagine that interest in personal disclosures and the sharing of secrets is a recent phenomenon. In fact, Ellenberger (1970) suggested that "pathogenic secrets"—those usually characterized by suppressed passion (jealousy, hatred, ambition), shame, or moral offense of a sexual nature—have been accorded a special place throughout history. Their importance, he noted, lies not in their content per se but in their meaning and dysfunctional consequences (e.g., anxiety, depression, impaired interpersonal relationships) among secret keepers. Ellenberger showed that, from the time of prehistory, there has been continued emphasis on the cathartic powers of revelation. The ritual of confession, implemented by early civilizations as well as by Catholic and some Protestant denominations, served as a precursor to modern psychological treatments that emphasize the need to reveal in order to heal. This is perhaps seen most profoundly in the orthodoxy of the Christian Church, which emphasizes the importance of, and even requires, confessing one's sins. Thus, keeping secrets, especially those that reflect acts, thoughts, or feelings of a forbidden nature, has long been associated with shame, guilt, and other forms of personal torment, while their disclosure has been linked with relief and exoneration.

A SHORT HISTORY OF SELF-DISCLOSURE RESEARCH

Research on self-disclosure in psychotherapy is, for the most part, a relatively recent (post-1990s) phenomenon, but research on the nature and processes of self-disclosure in everyday life has a longer history. The eminent social psychologist Kurt Lewin did some early (1948) work on disclosure, finding that Americans, in comparison to Germans, were more likely to be open, that is, to disclose private concerns, to strangers. The contemporary study of self-disclosure can essentially be traced to the work that Jourard began over 40 years ago (1964, 1968, 1971a, 1971b; Jourard & Lasakow, 1958). As part of his own existential quest, specifically his interest in finding out what it means to be a "real self," Jourard began studying lapses in understanding between people, a phenomenon he believed was at the root of problems in the family and in the greater society. His interest was spurred by the ideas of Fromm, Horney, and Riesman, all of whom, though employing different vocabularies, wrote about the deep sense of alienation they had observed in people and the tendency of most individuals to hide from or misrepresent themselves to others.

At roughly the same time, Goffman (1959), writing from a sociological perspective, introduced the enduring term "presentation of self in everyday life." According to both Goffman and Jourard, individuals' presentation or misrepresentation to others took a particular form, namely, attempting to represent oneself according to a "best-outcome" formula. That is, people seek to present themselves in a way that maximizes either others' views of them or, similarly, their own sense of fitting in well with the norms of the greater society. Genuineness, self-awareness, a need to be truly known by others—all were qualities seen to be essentially absent in the lives of post-World War II men and women. (See Richard Yates's great though overlooked classic 1961 novel on this theme, *Revolutionary Road*.) Furthermore, Goffman held that others colluded in this behavior; his sense was that part of what it means to be civilized is not to "steal" or actively pursue information that is not freely given to us.

Much of this perspective is strikingly similar to the British psychoanalyst D. W. Winnicott's (1960) notion of "false self." Winnicott posited that those who haven't been adequately nurtured early in life tend to present themselves in accord with the needs of others, a strategy adopted in a desperate attempt to please those upon whom one is dependent for love and affirmation. Individuals who have developed a stronger "false self" than "true self" are largely incapable of understanding, accepting, or acting in accord with their own needs. As a result, their interpersonal relationships are often strained and distant. Like Winnicott, Jourard was acutely aware of many individuals' avoidance of genuine intimacy with others, a tendency that at least partly reflected a fear of revealing themselves to others.

Jourard's work, then, falls somewhere along the intersection of social psychology ("How do we present ourselves to others?"), clinical psychology ("How do we relate to others and with what consequences for mental health?"), and existential psychology ("What does it mean to be genuine or real in life?"). In one of his first attempts to study these issues, he asked his friends a seemingly straightforward question: "What do you know about me?" He reported (1971b) that he "hardly recognized" himself from these answers, that his friends seemed not to know him at all. We might now see his surprise as somewhat naive—that is, he seemed to have taken his friends' responses at face value and seemed not to have factored in his friends' tact, honesty, or presentation of self, nor his own potential experimenter bias (i.e., that he might well have been looking to confirm his belief that others did not know him well and therefore remembered comments that confirmed his hypothesis more than comments that contradicted his hypothesis). Nevertheless, Jourard used this exercise to begin devising a list of questions that people often ask others in trying to forge personal relationships with them. After some tinkering, this list came to be the first version of what was to be the most widely used instrument in the field for several decades, "The Self-Disclosure Questionnaire" (Jourard & Lasakow, 1958).

Jourard came to believe that self-disclosure was central to an individual's mental health and a prerequisite for satisfying relationships with others. In fact, he suggested that not only was mental health contingent upon self-disclosure but that mental illness resulted from its absence: "When we succeed in hiding our being from others, we tend to lose touch with our real selves" (1971b, p. viii). Thus, Jourard contended that healthy people are those who are able to disclose themselves in some optimal degree to at least one significant other. Similarly, he held that the process of self-disclosure was critical to the development of intimate relationships and was associated, for example, with good marital adjustment. He believed that self-disclosure was facilitated by feelings of love and trust. If I love another, reasoned Jourard, I want him or her to know me as fully as possible; indeed, I show my love by striving to make this happen. However, Jourard's research revealed some surprises:

> One expects people to be transparent within the family, but we find much evidence of dissembling, of lack of mutual disclosure. Children do not know their parents, fathers do not know what their children think, or what they are doing. Husbands and wives often are strangers one to the other to an incredible degree. (p. 6)

One of Jourard's points of emphasis, one supported by research, is that disclosure is facilitated by reciprocity. Most individuals hold to the principle of disclosing to the same approximate degree that they are being disclosed to, a point nicely illustrated by Billy Joel's lyrics in the song "The Stranger": "Why were you surprised that you never saw the stranger/did you ever let your lover see the stranger in yourself?" Indeed, Jourard found that when reciprocity does not occur—when one member of a dyad discloses more than the other, or even senses this to be the case—conflict often results. This, of course, is a fairly typical pattern of marital conflict, most often represented by the wife's complaint that her husband does not share enough of his personal thoughts. For the most part, though, disclosure begets disclosure.

It takes courage to be self-revealing, to be truly known to others. "Man," observed Jourard, was the "master of the mendacious arts" (1971b, p. 17). Why we dissemble, why we keep secrets, why we stay hidden are questions that will be pursued throughout this book. Jourard had essentially two answers to these questions. One was that we have been handed down, often by religious leaders, an intimidating script of what we ought to be like (reflected in the Bible, and in various religious traditions), and thus acknowledgment of deviation from this script engenders shame. A second answer, Jourard thought, derives from the fact that openness is frightening: "We camouflage our true being before others to protect ourselves against criticism or rejection" (p. vii). Here again the contention is that we have internalized standards of appropriate behavior and thoughts and that others' knowledge of our deviation from these standards may engender shame, or even rejection. Similarly, Jourard made the point that self-disclosure makes us vulnerable—that when others know us well they have information that may be used for their own personal gain; they may well take advantage of that which we have revealed to them.

In the past two decades, the work of James Pennebaker (1990, 1995, 1997, 2002) has dominated the field of self-disclosure. Pennebaker's research has yielded two primary sets of findings: that the general tendency to keep secrets is related to a variety of psychological and physiological consequences, including depression, anxiety, headaches, and intrusive thoughts about the secret (see also Larson & Chastain, 1990); and that disclosure, via writing about trauma and stress, can significantly alleviate such symptomatology. These ideas will be discussed in greater detail in subsequent chapters.

POSITIVE AND NEGATIVE EFFECTS
OF SELF-DISCLOSURE

To Jourard, self-disclosure has two primary and related functions: to better connect with others and to better understand the self. That is, self-disclosure works in the service of both intimacy and identity. Moreover, as noted above, these two functions are constantly interacting: we trust, we disclose, we are disclosed to, we feel closer to another, we open ourselves up more to explore self and other. "When a man discloses his experiences to another, fully, spontaneously, and honestly, then the mystery that he was decreases enormously. . . . Self disclosure between men reduces the mystery that one man is for another. It is the empirical index of the I–Thou relationship which I, agreeing with Buber, see as the index of man functioning at his highest and truly human level" (1971b, pp. 5–6). Here Jourard acclaims self-disclosure as an ideal, as a goal to strive for in our existential quest to be fully connected to others.

Others, including Pennebaker (1995) and Stiles (1987, 1995), have suggested that individuals also disclose to achieve catharsis (i.e., an emotional purging of long-suppressed feelings or even of recent traumatic events) and to determine the extent to which their behaviors, feelings, and thoughts are normative. However, the extent to which disclosure leads to catharsis and, relatedly, the extent to which it is helpful or harmful remain hotly contested issues in contemporary psychological thought that will be revisited throughout this volume.

There are, I believe, at least six positive aspects of self-disclosure, most of which overlap with those enumerated by Jourard and others. Here I will just note them briefly; in the next chapter, I'll elaborate on how they manifest in the context of psychotherapy.

1. Experiencing a greater sense of emotional closeness to another through sharing meaningful aspects of oneself (intimacy). Essentially: "When I speak with you this way, I feel close to you."
2. Being known and affirmed by another (validation and affirmation). Essentially: "Please let me know that what I did was right."
3. Gaining greater insight into oneself and gaining a more cohesive sense of self (insight and identity formation). Essentially: "As I reveal myself, I become clearer about who I am."
4. Expanding one's sense of self through the process of disclosing multiple aspects of self (differentiation of self). Essentially: "The more I disclose, the more I understand all the different parts of myself."
5. Achieving a greater sense of authenticity through acknowledging and sharing deeply personal aspects of oneself (authenticity). Essentially: "It feels so good to be honest in speaking with you."
6. Relieving the physiological and psychological pressures of painful and/or shameful experiences (catharsis). Essentially: "It's such a relief to get this off my chest."

In short, we disclose in order to feel closer to another, to feel validated by another, to understand and strengthen the core aspects of our identity, to explore and accept multiple aspects of ourselves, to feel more genuine in the world, and to relieve the burden of unexpressed pain.

Not surprisingly, many researchers and theorists believe we are better off when we open up, as disclosure is apparently good for both the body and soul. Indeed, some see virtually no "downside" to such behavior, regardless of the circumstances. This perspective assumes a rather simple "the more, the better" approach to disclosure. However, self-disclosure, like any other usually benign phenomenon (including psychotherapy), may also be painful and even harmful. A posting on the Internet cleverly limned the need to be prudent around self-disclosures: "There are two rules for success in life. Rule 1: Don't tell people everything you know."

Kowalski (1999) summarized the potential negative consequences of self-disclosure. Because these are not as easily imagined as the positive consequences, I'll provide brief descriptions below. Again, though, I'll discuss each in far greater detail in the next chapter, emphasizing how these potential outcomes play out in the realm of psychotherapy.

1. *Being rejected by the recipient of our disclosure.* In revealing a private part of ourselves, we ask another to accept this previously unknown aspect of ourselves. In doing so, we risk rejection. Jessica Benjamin (1994) suggested that to become known or recognized is immediately to experience the other's power: "The other becomes the one who can . . . see what is hidden; who can reach, conceivably even violate, the core of the self" (p. 539). Sometimes the recipient of our disclosure doesn't explicitly reject or shame us but rather takes the opportunity to propound endlessly on his or her vaguely similar predicament or accomplishments. When others "rain on our parade," it is so very hurtful.

2. *Burdening another with our secrets.* We face the risk of burdening others with our secrets or thoughts. For example, I may not choose to share with a friend or family member that I am distressed if I believe that he or she will lose sleep over this, feel responsible for doing something about it, or identify too strongly with the source of my pain. Furthermore, I may not share some accomplishment if I feel that the other person will be burdened by competitive or envious feelings. Tact often stands in dialectical opposition to the dictates of full disclosure.

3. *Creating undesired impressions about ourselves.* Related to the risk of rejection is the possibility of being seen differently, less positively, as a consequence of disclosure. Some individuals are capable of accepting another "warts and all." Others, however, may struggle to incorporate new, unpleasant information into a long-standing image. A good illustration of this is contained in the lyrics of Carly Simon's song "We Have No Secrets." Her words in the song suggest that, although she knows her lover better when he shares his past, the price paid for the knowledge is too high. Indeed, she laments, it's often better never to have known these secrets at all.

4. *Feeling regret for not having shared the secret earlier.* Kowalski (1999) proposed that the timing of disclosures can cause regret. We become aware that we could have, perhaps should have, brought this issue up

before. We realize that we have been living with a lie, or at least with thoughts or feelings that have been unexpressed. Why we waited so long is a question that can cause a good deal of self-doubt, especially when the recipient of our disclosure responds with acceptance or compassion.

5. *Experiencing increased vulnerability.* Intimate disclosure may upset our personal boundaries—we feel we have given away too much of ourselves and feel vulnerable as a consequence. In fact, there is substantial evidence (see Hoyt, 1978) to support the idea that secret keeping contributes to a coherent sense of self, one that is experienced as separate, unique, and powerful. Some individuals are comfortable with openness and personal disclosure; others prefer, indeed need, to stay relatively closed and non-disclosing. The point is that some disclosures may make some individuals feel shaky, somewhat unwound, and needing to rapidly close up in order to feel safe again.

6. *Experiencing a sense of shame following acknowledgment of thoughts, feelings, or deeds that are discrepant with our ideal sense of self.* The most often cited negative consequence of disclosure (one that permeates all other noted dysfunctional effects) is that of personal shame. In disclosing aspects of myself that I fear others will not accept, I am also forced to face those unwanted parts of myself. The pride I may feel in owning up to past mistakes or adopting a view of myself that includes elements of disillusionment or disappointment may be balanced by the discomfiture of realizing that I am not the person I wish to be. These thoughts, of course, may arise in the privacy of my own consciousness. But shame at who I am or what I have done is inevitably exacerbated by disclosure to others.

MISUSES OF DISCLOSURE

Disclosures are most often thought of as positive events; even the negative consequences noted above tend to be thought of as unfortunate by-products of courageous acts. Moreover, research has shown that high disclosers tend to be thought of as friendly, open, and approachable (Collins & Miller, 1994). But there are exceptions to these general principles because disclosures are not always used in the service of growth or intimacy or healing. Rather, some disclosures seem to be in the service of distancing from or controlling or hurting others. Because disclosures are necessarily selective—at any one time we typically have multiple and competing feelings and thoughts—we are almost always in a position of deciding at any given moment whether and what to disclose. I could disclose to a friend that I am tired, thus effectively distancing us at the moment, and while this feeling might be somewhat true, it also likely represents one of many possible responses, including perhaps, "I'm still feeling sad [or overwhelmed or preoccupied] about something that I want to share with you." A friend of mine acknowledges that in dating situations she often shares some unfavorable aspect of herself as a way of inhibiting further intimacy.

Derlega, Metts, Petronio, and Margulis (1993) offer an example of a disclosure that is controlling: "Most of us have had the experience of getting into a conversation with someone who begins to tell us very personal things about him- or herself. If we are not interested in developing a relationship with this person, we may feel uncomfortable. Perhaps without being aware of it, we are responding to the unspoken assumption that we too will divulge personal information when we really do not want to" (p. 3). That is, sometimes disclosures may be used in a manipulative fashion to attempt to get personal information, such as gossip, from another.

Some disclosures serve to drive wedges among group or family members. This occurs when some members in a group or family are privy to the secret while others are not. The notion of "triangulation," so essential to family therapy, offers a means of understanding this dynamic. In the "family secret triangle," the teller of the secret ("the silencer"), those bound to keep the secret ("the silenced"), and those who are uninformed each face a unique predicament that compromises open communication and integrity within the family dynamic (Institute for Mental Health Initiatives, 1995). For the silencer, fear of exposure and feelings of guilt and shame can often produce as much anxiety as the keeping of the secret was intended to control. Those who are silenced may experience a loss of self-respect for keeping the secret but may fear recrimination or rejection if they tell. Those who are uninformed, in turn, become isolated in their ignorance and unable to make decisions about their own lives because they are missing important information.

Another misuse of disclosure, and one that we have probably all been subject to, occurs when a person is intent on dominating a conversation, forcing us to listen to endless stories of his or her exploits, achievements, or complaints. The disclosures of people with narcissistic, borderline, or other personality disorders are frequently not in the service of intimacy but rather in the service of using others to satisfy self needs.

Similarly, disclosures are aversive when the frequency of disclosures surrounding hurt or angry feelings greatly exceeds disclosures of benevolent or affectionate feelings. Partners who are more apt to share hurt feelings or critical thoughts of the other are self-disclosing in a skewed way. This imbalance will inevitably have consequences for the relationship. In general, knowing when, where, what, and how to disclose to an intimate partner—that is, knowing how to be tactful—is a great asset to the relationship. As many researchers of intimate relationships have pointed out, total and complete honesty is not only impossible in a relationship, it is usually not even desirable. What comes to mind here is the cartoon in which the husband says to the wife: "If you ask me one more time what's wrong, I'm going to tell you."

DECIDING TO DISCLOSE:
THE EXPRESSION–REPRESSION DEBATE

> "[R]epression is totally false and mechanical. Everybody knows that. We're not supposed to deny our nature."
> "It's natural to deny our nature. . . . It's the whole point of being different from animals."
> "But that's crazy."
> "It's the only way to survive."
> —DeLillo (1985, p. 296)

Given the multiple positive and negative consequences of disclosure, it is often extremely difficult for individuals to decide whether and what to reveal to others. Indeed, although disclosure of painful material has been the cornerstone of psychotherapy since its inception, in recent years there have been numerous challenges to the idea that "getting things out in the open" is simply the best, or most psychologically healthy, strategy. Many researchers point to the value of repression in certain circumstances—the very thing Freud cautioned against so strongly.

For example, Kelly and McKillop (1996) contend that secrets should be revealed only when the keeper is particularly troubled by the secret and/or when the confidant(e) is likely to react positively to the revelation. "Although confessions may be 'good for the soul,' given that they can wreak havoc with one's network of friends and supporters, some things truly are better left unsaid" (p. 461). They advise people to scrutinize their friends and relations for their ability to keep the secret and to offer new insights without being judgmental.

Bernard Kempler, a Polish survivor of the Holocaust, has written compellingly about the tension between expression and repression of traumatic memories. In order to survive, he was forced to conceal his true identity, assuming a false name, a feminine disguise, a false religion, and fictional parents. While Kempler admits that his childhood experiences were atypical, he holds that most, if not all, people have grown up with some good reason to hide parts of their true selves. "While actual survival may not be at stake, the survival of some part—a way of feeling, a certain individual inclination or a way of perceiving, an impulse, a desire, an imaginative turn, an inspiration—may have been threatened with serious devaluation or even extinction" (1987, p. 111). Uncritical self-disclosure, he suggests, can be harmful to ourselves and others. Kempler speaks of responsible self-disclosure as that which greatly "differs from mental incontinence, a giving in to an impulse to blurt out uncritically what has become difficult to hold in" (p. 114).

While Kempler takes a moderate position in the expression–repression debate, others have been far more adamant about the need to forget—to suppress distressing thoughts and feelings—in order to move on. Joyce Carol Oates expressed such sentiments in an article about the events of September 11:

> As soon as [a tragic] experience is over, we begin the inevitable process of "healing": that is, forgetting. We extract from the helpless visceral sensation some measure of intellectual summary or control. We lie to ourselves: we revise experience to make it lighthearted and amusing to others. For in what other way is terror to be tamed, except recycled as anecdotes or aphorisms, a sugary coating to hide the bitter pellet of truth within? (2001, p. A11)

A fair amount of empirical evidence has also been offered in support of the long-term value of repression and other mechanisms of denial. While repressors (those who tend to push distressing thoughts and, even more so, distressing feelings out of awareness) may incur some physical costs (e.g., increased somatic complaints), they tend to have fewer psychological symptoms over time than do nonrepressors (Bonanno, Keltner, Holen, & Horowitz, 1995). For example, individuals who are more emotionally avoidant during bereavement have better long-term adaptation (Bonanno et al., 1995). Conversely, those who disclose emotions either verbally or in written form do not manifest better adjustment in recovering from the death of a spouse (Stroebe, Stroebe, Schut, Zech, & van den Bout, 2002). Furthermore, patients with a repressive coping style manifest fewer symptoms of acute stress disorder and posttraumatic stress disorder following heart attacks than do nonrepressors (Ginzberg, Solomon, & Bleich, 2002). Bonanno (2004) has argued that there are multiple pathways to resilience, including repressive coping, overly positive self-bias, and a sense of personal hardiness—all of which obviate the need to talk about traumatic experiences.

Clearly, there is no "right answer" to the question of whether repressing or expressing emotions or thoughts leads to better outcomes. Disclosure often reduces symptoms in the long term but may lead to short-term distress (Smyth, 1998); moreover, it is unlikely to be helpful if it takes the form of repetitive reviews of details and feelings (Nolen-Hoeksema, McBride, & Larson, 1997). As Pennebaker (cited in Murray, 2002) has indicated, "People who [write] about things over and over in the same ways aren't getting any better. There has to be growth or change in the way they view their experiences" (p. 55).

Moreover, the value of disclosure is likely to be a function of individual differences: Repression may be more beneficial for repressors, while disclosure may be especially beneficial for nonrepressors. Still, even this seemingly simple formulation is complicated by the fact that repressors and nonrepressors are better thought of as existing on a continuum rather than as strict categories. Individuals may act different ways at different times or even evidence some combination of both tendencies at the same time. Recently, Bonanno, Papa, O'Neill, Westphal, and Coifman (2004) found that those New York City college students who were able to both express and suppress their emotions on command were those who experienced the least distress a year and a half after the 9/11 attacks. Thus, at least in the aftermath of specific trauma, the ability to be cognitively flexible—to be able to express as well as repress emotions—may be a more effective strategy than adherence to only one of these positions. In short, assessing the value of disclosure is an extremely complex problem. This issue will be further explored in Chapter 4 in the context of a discussion of when and whether disclosure in psychotherapy is helpful.

Given the potential benefits and drawbacks of self-disclosure, the maxim of many secret-keepers indeed might be "To tell or not to tell—that is the question." Larson (1993) notes that "there is often an ambivalent, approach-avoidance quality to our experience in these moments" (p. 97). At the heart of the conflict is the desire to maintain one's self-esteem: Though we may long to be close to another and share parts of ourselves, the resulting vulnerability and shame may be more than we can bear. Thus, those who harbor intimate personal information face the question of whether to retain this knowledge in their hearts and minds, locking it impenetrably within, or whether to reveal this information, thereby transforming it into something acknowledged, shared, and stored in more than one body and mind.

What are the major lessons therapists may learn from this wealth of new information regarding interpersonal disclosure? First, that despite its positive functions, disclosure is fraught with significant psychological risks that therapists must heed. Second, and relatedly, individuals differ significantly in their willingness to disclose and the benefits they derive in doing so. And finally, the norms surrounding disclosure in this country have changed dramatically during the past few decades. While there are great individual differences, many patients have grown up in a "confessional culture," disclosing personal issues to an extent unheard-of in previous generations, and many will expect a significant degree of self-disclosure from their therapists. These issues and other topics related to patient disclosure will be explored in greater detail in the next chapter.

CHAPTER 2

Clinical Perspectives
on Patient Disclosure

I suppose one never does tell anybody everything about oneself.
Except one's analyst of course.
                                              —LODGE (1995, p. 140)

Disclosure is at the heart of psychotherapy.
                                              —STILES (1995, p. 71)

As the previous chapter noted, disclosure in therapy has become a prominent and controversial issue in recent years, with articles and professional
conferences on this theme abounding. Most of this work has focused on
therapist disclosure to patients, as psychodynamically oriented clinicians in
particular have struggled over the appropriateness, benefits, and implications of sharing their thoughts, feelings, and even personal issues with their
patients.

Nevertheless, the original clinical interest in disclosure focused squarely
on the patient, not the therapist. Freud urged his patients to speak freely, to tell
him whatever was on their mind regardless of how insignificant or shameful it
might appear ("the fundamental rule"). Early clinical innovations—from free
association, to lying on the couch, to the therapist's silence and neutrality
("blank screen")—were justified as facilitating the patient's ability to reveal
thoughts without censorship. Discovering that despite his best efforts patients could not or would not speak openly, Freud's attention expanded from
the nature of patients' disclosures to the reasons they could not disclose, that
is, their resistance to speaking freely and openly to him. Following Freud, the
analytic community continued to focus its attention on these and related issues, theorizing on such topics as the meaning of silence, the importance of

letting the patient begin sessions, the keeping of secrets, and the characteristic ways that certain types of patients avoid therapeutic engagement and disclosure. Anna Freud (1958), for example, suggested that adolescents experience particular difficulties in being forthcoming with their analysts because of their need to feel absolutely independent of any authority figure who reminds them of their parents. During the past decade or so, a number of researchers (e.g., Farber, 2003; Hill, Thompson, & Corbett, 1992; Kelly, 1998, 2000; Stiles, 1995) have begun to empirically address issues relating to patient disclosure.

It is also important to keep in mind that, despite the recent upsurge of interest in the topic of therapist disclosure, the shape and focus of clinical sessions are typically far more affected by the nature, manner, and extent of patient disclosures. Thus, before turning to the more widely addressed phenomenon of therapist disclosure, several aspects of patient disclosure will be addressed in the next few chapters. This chapter reviews a wide range of clinical issues: the extent to which verbal disclosure is emphasized in different therapeutic models; the nature and importance of nonverbal disclosure; factors affecting disclosure, including legal rulings; positive and negative consequences of disclosure; and therapists' responses to disclosure. My interjections in this chapter (and others in the book) reflect my own bias: that, despite the problems inherent in disclosure, the benefits substantially outweigh the pitfalls for most individuals. Thus, I believe that, in general, patients should be encouraged to disclose (albeit at their own pace) and that therapists, supervisors, and supervisees should also self-disclose (prudently), especially around "process" issues—the interpersonal stuff that is happening in the room at the moment. Like Stiles (1995), I am convinced that disclosure is at the heart of psychotherapeutic (and supervisory) matters. A great deal of healing and intimacy begins with the words "Let's talk about it."

PATIENT DISCLOSURE ACROSS DIFFERENT THEORETICAL MODELS OF THERAPY

For many patients the therapist's office is, indeed, the place where they disclose their most intimate thoughts, speaking of things they would not share with friends, lovers, family, or clergy. Some come to therapy expressly for this reason—to speak of what has been previously unspeakable, to unburden themselves of long-kept secrets. All therapists have observed the great anxiety in new patients as they sit down for the first session and begin revealing the details of experiences or feelings that have been kept private for so long. And all have also witnessed the great relief many of these patients experience, even with little or no intervention on the therapist's part (save perhaps for active listening). More than any specific benefit, though, patient disclosure provides the data for the therapist's understanding and clinical interventions.

But, of course, the process is not quite this simple. As was described in the preceding chapter, disclosure poses danger, especially of shame. Moreover, even those patients who are more influenced by the positive aspects of disclosure than by the negative—who are highly motivated to disclose and trusting of their therapist—may well be confronted with the realization that full disclosure is more of an ideal to be pursued than an actual possibility. What could it even mean? At any given moment, there are myriad choices of what to address, including feelings about one's therapist, thoughts about last week's session, dreams, events that occurred in one's childhood, and the latest fight or misunderstanding with one's spouse, boss, friend, child, or parent. Inevitably, the patient must choose what to disclose and, in doing so, he or she necessarily chooses not to disclose the infinite universe of other thoughts and feelings.

The theoretical model adopted by the therapist exerts a considerable influence on the process and content of patient disclosure. Clearly, the press to reveal one's innermost thoughts is most evident in psychodynamically oriented therapy, wherein the methods (e.g., interpretations) and goals of treatment (e.g., increased self-awareness) are inextricably connected to disclosures. Therapists working within this and related (e.g., Jungian) traditions value and foster patients' explorations of increasingly deep, personally revealing material. Indeed, such approaches have also been known as "insight-oriented" therapies, reflecting the fact that the work primarily involves a patient's ability to learn and change through revealing and understanding past patterns of behavior. The therapist's task is to encourage disclosure (even at times by remaining silent) and point out resistances to it. The assumption within the psychodynamic model is that disclosures will become deeper as therapy progresses, as the therapeutic alliance is strengthened, as resistances are confronted and worked through, and as useful insights emerge. Contemporary forms of psychodynamic treatment, often grouped under the rubric of relational therapy, place a greater emphasis than traditional models on the importance of both participants in therapy being fully open about the ongoing process that is unfolding between them. Thus, patient disclosure in this model of therapy is as much about revealing here-and-now feelings and thoughts as it is about revealing events of the past.

Other therapies are more ambiguous regarding the necessity of client self-disclosure and the therapist's responsibility for facilitating it. For example, humanistic therapy holds that clients will become more open and disclosing in response to the therapist's ability to be disclosing (what Rogers called "transparent"), empathic, and positively regarding. According to Rogers (1957), these are the "necessary and sufficient" conditions of therapy and, if provided, lead inevitably to patient growth, self-awareness, and self-actualization. But Rogers did not believe that a client needed to delve deeply into past material and did not push clients either in that direction or in the direction of discussing transferential feelings. In fact, he was upbraided by the analytic community for being superficial in his approach. It is probably unfair to label Rogers in this manner—videotapes and transcripts of his sessions reveal clients disclosing a great deal about issues of current importance and their here-and-now feelings toward Rogers himself, apparently in response to Rogers' extraordinarily gentle and accepting manner (Farber, Brink, & Raskin, 1996). Still, it is true that his work is not predicated on the need for clients to go deeply into the past or to explore the nature and meaning of complex and intense feelings in the room.

Therapists utilizing cognitive therapy (CT) or cognitive-behavioral therapy (CBT) models are, somewhat paradoxically, even more active than psychodynamically oriented therapists in pursuing their clients' underlying assumptions and values (schemas), but their goals generally do not include the progressive uncovering of childhood memories or creating meaning out of disparate elements of what is uncovered. They do not adhere to classical psychoanalysts' "onion" model of disclosure, wherein the task is to peel away progressive layers of thoughts and memories till the raw, primitive indications of sex, aggression, and childhood experiences emerge. Instead, they tend to focus on identifying and altering current maladaptive patterns of thoughts, feelings, and behaviors.

Moreover, whereas psychodynamically oriented therapies emphasize and encourage disclosure of traumatic material and dysphoric affect as a means of understanding and working through these experiences, CBT favors the relatively rapid displacement of troubling, negatively tinged schemas with more positive thoughts. Psychodynamically oriented therapies thus favor a "tragic" vision of reality, one rooted in elements of ambiguity, complexity, and the inevitable harshness of life; by contrast, behavioral and cognitive-behavioral therapies favor a "comic" vision of reality, one that emphasizes control, predictability, and the possibility of successfully resolving difficult problems (Messer & Winokur, 1980). This essential difference in philosophy necessarily affects the nature of disclosure in these therapeutic approaches. Although no study has yet investigated differences in patient disclosure as a function of therapeutic modalities, it is likely that disclosures in CBT, relative to those in dynamically oriented therapy, would be of lesser breadth (fewer issues disclosed) and depth (less extensive focus on any given issue, at least in terms of discussion of the etiology or personal meaning of symptoms). Such putative differences, of course, may be entirely unrelated to differences in therapeutic outcome, especially if outcome is defined in terms of symptom reduction rather than self-understanding. Furthermore, there is certainly considerable variation among therapists adhering to any theoretical tradition in regard to what each prefers his or her patients to discuss.

Most importantly, though, what must be kept in mind is that, even within therapies that do not emphasize the value of revealing deeper aspects of self nor here-and-now feelings toward the therapist, patients invariably disclose private details of their lives. The material in all verbally mediated therapies, the stuff that therapists and patients work with, typically consists of those aspects of self that are difficult to share with others and may even be difficult to acknowledge to oneself.

PATIENT DISCLOSURE IN GROUP THERAPY

The complex web of interpersonal relationships within a group therapy setting complicates greatly the nature and process of individual disclosure. The critical tension here is between the increased potential for shame—because one is revealing in front of a group—and the increased pull for disclosure as a result of the power of group cohesion, support, and norms. In some ways, then, disclosure in groups is more frightening for many individuals even as it affords an especially powerful way of being cared for and emotionally held by multiple others.

The structure of group therapy leads to possibilities of distrusting the group leader, of fearing for one's emotional safety, and of doubting the confidentiality of the group. In addition, groups afford individuals more hiding places than individual therapy and greater opportunities for relative anonymity. That is, a group member may allow others to disclose while he or she remains more or less hidden. In fact, the group dynamics may operate in a way that makes some individuals designated disclosers and others listeners. The manifestation of any of these dynamics can lead to too little or too superficial disclosure on the part of group members. Group therapy can also lead to group members' vying for the attention and approval of the therapist, a situation that may result in some members increasing the frequency or intensity of their disclosures.

Group therapy patients who disclose too little or too much may alienate other members who are not prepared to disclose in a reciprocal manner. However, a well-functioning group with a savvy leader is likely to become aware of these dynamics and, while respecting individual differences regarding frequency or depth of disclosure, attempt to re-engage those group members who disclosures have fallen below group norms and inhibit those group members who tend to monopolize group time.

Vinogradov and Yalom (1990) have suggested that an importance difference between disclosure in group and individual therapy is a greater emphasis on horizontal or here-and-now disclosures in the group situation. That is, in group therapy, the discussion tends to revolve around patients' (and therapists') immediate thoughts, feelings, and reactions to other group members. Slavin (1993), in fact, found that only here-and-now disclosures predicted group cohesion, a factor considered to be critical for effective group therapy (Yalom, 1970) and for members' individual growth (Tschuschke & Dies, 1997). My own sense is that disclosure in group therapy is particularly effective—and especially appropriate for those with deficits in interpersonal functioning—because it combines some of the best features of contemporary individual psychodynamic therapy and CBT. That is, disclosure in group therapy involves frequent processing of thoughts and feelings, especially those that are interpersonally related, and often results in immediate feedback and advice regarding what is dysfunctional and in what directions these thoughts and feelings should be modified.

NONVERBAL SELF-DISCLOSURE

He that has eyes to see and ears to hear may convince himself that no mortal can keep a secret. If his lips are silent, he chatters with his fingertips; betrayal oozes out of him at every pore.
—FREUD (1905, p. 215)

Although verbal self-disclosure is the primary focus of this chapter, it is clear that patients can also express themselves through nonverbal means. In fact, many let their therapists know that they "don't have the words for this" or can only "partially say this in words." Ekman's work on facial expressions (e.g., Ekman & Rosenberg, 1998) reminds us that we miss so much about others by attending to words alone and that, in fact, such attention can obscure important data. For example, Bonanno and colleagues (2002) found that, in comparison to survivors of childhood sexual abuse who had disclosed their experiences, nondisclosers showed significantly greater nonverbal expression of shame during an opportunity to disclose these experiences. "What cannot be said will get wept" noted the seventh-century poet Sappho (cited in Harrison, 2004, p. 13).

Within the category of nonverbal behavior, a distinction may be made between nonverbal expression that has been explicitly elicited by the therapist (such as a picture in art therapy or a dance movement) and nonverbal expression that is embedded in a patient's demeanor and behavior, including facial expressions, eye contact, posture, laughter, tears, and vocal inflections. In the former case, nonverbal expression is the purpose and primary activity of the therapy and typically results in a product or performance of some kind. The latter type reflects a broader phenomenon, one that is powerful and noteworthy despite its relative neglect in therapies that emphasize the value of spoken language. For example, "acting-out" behavior (e.g., maintaining silence, grimacing, arm-folding, walking around a therapist's office) may become the predominant narrative for some patients in some sessions. More generally, nonverbal expression constitutes a virtually ubiquitous aspect of clients' overall presentation, and as such is an invaluable source of clinical information.

Some nonverbal behaviors consistently, though not unfailingly, reflect a particular emotional state. A patient's welling up with tears typically indicates sadness, while fidgeting is usually an indicator of anxiety. Smiling, as noted in a classic rock song ("Wooden Ships") by Crosby, Stills, and Nash, is virtually a universal signal of warmth and acceptance. But most nonverbal behaviors require careful attention to such contextual factors as the patient's characteristic interpersonal style and the nature of the therapeutic relationship. A patient who rarely meets the therapist's gaze during a session may be characterologically avoidant but may also "simply" be absorbed in thought, experiencing discomfort or anger with the therapist or the therapy process, or feeling comfortable enough in the room to allow his or her gaze to roam. Ultimately, in an undertaking as complex and interpersonally situated as therapy—and one in which agreement around the meaning of words and gestures is so very important—hypotheses based on nonverbal cues invariably require further testing in the verbal realm.

Many therapists do, in fact, attend carefully to nonverbal cues as a means of understanding what the patent may be feeling but unable to express verbally. Experienced therapists in particular are often able to identify anxiety or sadness as soon as a patient enters the office, and are probably at least as likely to glean early manifestations of resistance or angry or erotic feelings from nonverbal behavior as from direct verbal expression. Furthermore, some therapeutic models emphasize a quite explicit focus on a patient's nonverbal cues. In Gestalt therapy, therapist attention to discrepancies between patient verbal and nonverbal expression is considered an integral aspect of the therapeutic process. And in short-term dynamic psychotherapy (McCullough et al., 2003), recognition of affect through nonverbal expression is an important aspect of the treatment. For example, the therapist must be able to distinguish between a "fake smile of serenity," and "genuine relaxation and enjoyment" (McCullough et al., 2003, p. 123). The therapist's attunement to nuances of nonverbal affective expression enables him or her to guide the patient toward more adaptive and authentic modes of expression.

Psychodynamically oriented therapists have also occasionally taken their cue from Freud in observing both verbal and nonverbal expressions of affect. The therapist's attunement to nonverbal cues is seen as helpful in gaining insight into the patient's dynamics and intrapsychic conflict. Mahl (1977)—who for years taught the Freud course at Yale University—recounts the story of "Mrs. B," who, while discussing her inferiority feelings as a wife and homemaker, placed her fingers over her mouth for a moment:

> Three minutes later she was saying, *spontaneously*, that her feelings of inferiority dated from her childhood. Then she had felt she was homely

and not as pretty as her sister, because she then had *two ugly protruding front teeth*. We inferred that the slight action of putting her fingers to her mouth anticipated, and perhaps facilitated, this recollection and verbalization about her childhood buckteeth. (p. 292, emphasis in original)

Mahl suggests that these kinds of observations on the part of the therapist can help to address one of Freud's essential questions: How does the unconscious become conscious? Still, these exceptions aside, insight-oriented therapists have devoted most of their theoretical, clinical, and research attention to what patients do and do not say. Geller (2005) is surely right in advocating for therapists to attend more carefully to stylistic elements of patients' clinical presentation.

Interdisciplinary lines of research have focused on the origins of nonverbal communication in ways that may inform our knowledge of the therapeutic encounter. Schore (2000), for example, has described the early development and maintenance of what he terms a "nonverbal affect lexicon"—a "vocabulary for nonverbal affective signals such as facial expressions, gestures, and vocal tone or prosody" (p. 31). An effective therapist, Schore implies, is one who interprets, reciprocates, and fosters the healthy growth of patients' nonverbal affective behavior.

Work done on affective communication via facial expression may also further our understanding of the effective ingredients of therapeutic work. Anstadt, Merten, Ullrich, and Krause (1997) studied the affective facial behavior of therapists and patients and found that compensatory, not reciprocal, affective facial behavior of the therapist is related to treatment success. A compensatory affective reaction might be a display of negative affect while the patient is denying negative affect through a display of facial happiness. Reciprocity, on the other hand, as in mutually displayed "happiness," is likely a "consequence of a mutual defense pattern centered around affective denial of the problems the patient is offering" (p. 413). The implication is that the therapist's reciprocal facial expression may reinforce and thus serve to maintain maladaptive relationship patterns, whereas compensatory facial expression may facilitate their cessation. As potentially important as this research is, much further work is needed in this area before we accept these finding as definitive. Not only are these findings somewhat counterintuitive in their refutation of empathic nonverbal responses on the part of the therapist, but also they overlook the potential critical influence of individual differences based on variables ranging from patient diagnosis to the strength of the therapeutic alliance.

In one of the few direct studies of nonverbal behavior in psychotherapy, Johnson, Geller, and Rhodes (1994) found that patients' feelings of being misunderstood by the therapist were often manifest nonverbally. They found that patients' gestures (arm or hand movements directly tied to speech) decreased from before to during those occasions on which they felt their therapist did not "really get" what they meant (p. 55). The authors speculated that misunderstandings have a devitalizing effect, such that deficits in nonverbal behaviors—a kind of motoric deflation—seem to result. Again, although these findings are provocative and heuristically valuable, they are based on a very small sample (six patients and six therapists) and are perhaps best thought of as preliminary evidence of a direct link between misunderstandings and nonverbal behavior in the therapy room.

THERAPIES THAT ARE PREDOMINANTLY NONVERBAL

Greater attention to nonverbal communication in traditional talk therapies seems indicated, but, as noted above, the emphasis in these therapies has generally been on verbal aspects of therapist–client interaction. There are, however, certain types of therapy that are based explicitly upon patients' self-disclosure through nonverbal means. These treatments, often referred to as "expressive therapies," utilize the media of art, music, psychodrama, movement, or dance in conjunction with, or in lieu of, a traditional talking therapy. While the theoretical underpinnings of these practices reside within diverse orientations—from the strictly psychological to the artistic and spiritual—their commonality lies in two primary assumptions: that there is something of therapeutic value to be derived from overt nonverbal expression; and that this expression can tap into psychological material that may not be accessible otherwise (i.e., through verbal means).

From the perspective of art, dance, or movement therapists, clients are seen as embodying their feelings or impulses. The therapist's task, therefore, is to concretize this in a way that makes clients more present, conscious, and accepting of who they are and what they are thinking or feeling. For example, a client who is walking intensely, with teeth clenched, might be seen by the therapist as harboring unexpressed aggression. The therapist, then, might help the client openly express these feelings through movement, for example, by having the client walk faster or stronger, which in turn may lead to stamping feet, clenching fists, and punching. Expressed aggression may evolve into assertiveness, an increased awareness of self, and an ability to stand firm with confidence.

Dance/movement therapy taps into the mind–body connection by encouraging clients to use movement as a form of expression. In her (2002) book *Offering from the Conscious Body*, Janet Adler describes authentic movement (one form of dance/movement therapy), emphasizing the study of "immediate" experience and the way in which a description of one's movement may take the place of naming complex, raw emotions. In this passage, she writes of the conclusion of a particular session with a client:

I see tears spilling from the mover's eyes as she speaks. The space between and around us suddenly deepens as we sit together, looking at each other, both receiving her simple and truthful words. Because of the way in which she speaks these words, opening to the fullness of her moving experience, she is filling with emotion. . . . These movement words glisten as the bare bones of what we come to know later as a source of deep suffering. (p. 16)

Here the "product" open to interpretation and exploration is bodily movement, in contrast to the more tangible, less transitory, art object or, even more typically, memories and thoughts. Thus, dance/movement therapy places its emphasis on immediate experience, which lends itself to considerable freedom of symbolic interpretation on the part of both therapist and client. Authentic movement, says Adler, allows an individual to find her way toward "speaking that which her body knows" (p. 16).

Another form of expressive therapy is play therapy, a modality grounded in the analogy that play is to children as words are to adults. In play therapy, children may express complex emotions that they would otherwise be unable to relate through words; they may also act out emotions and behaviors that might not be considered acceptable in "real life," and then be guided in examining them. Children may be able to project "unacceptable" emotions (for example, sadness or anger) or behavior (for example, physical or sexual abuse) that they could not or would not be able to verbally articulate onto inanimate objects such as dolls.

VARIABLES INFLUENCING PATIENT TENDENCY TO DISCLOSE

In addition to considerations of therapeutic orientation and modality, several other factors may affect patients' willingness to disclose in therapy. An awareness of these factors should enable therapists to better judge the extent to which patients can or should be encouraged to modify the breadth or depth of their disclosures.

The Patient's Comfort Level in Revealing Stressful Material

As a consequence of biological, familial, and/or cultural influences, some patients are especially prone to concealing even moderately personal information (Coates & Winston, 1987; Kahn, Achter, & Shambaugh, 2001; Larson & Chastain, 1990; Macdonald & Morley, 2001; Mikulincer & Nachson, 1991). For such individuals, the sharing of personal information with anyone, especially those outside the family constellation, is antithetical to their temperament and to long-standing deeply held values. By contrast, other patients are surprisingly open to disclosing seemingly intensely shameful material. This may be a consequence of having grown up in a very open family, being securely attached as a child, attending therapy previously, having a strong positive sense of self, or being part of a strong supportive social network (Hessling & Kahn, 2000). Kahn et al. (2001) use the term "distress disclosure" to refer to the general tendency of individuals to disclose (vs. conceal) personally distressing information.

In a related vein (see Chapter 1), patients who are primarily "sensitizers" are aware of and need to discuss painful aspects of their environment; by contrast, "repressors" tend to disavow stressful stimuli and seemingly have little or no need to talk about such events. Clearly, therapists need to be aware of a patient's "comfort zone" in terms of disclosure and adjust their own level of probing and challenging in response to what a patient can profitably accept.

The Extent to Which the Patient Feels the Issue Is Pressing and Urgent

Some patients come into therapy with an urgent need to discuss a particular issue. Their symptoms, most often connected to anxiety or depression, feel overwhelming, and as a result they seem virtually compelled to speak openly about this problem. On the other end of the continuum are those who enter therapy without having fully "owned" their need to be there and thus seem reluctant to delve deeply into the heart of any matter. Often these are individuals who are in therapy on the advice or urging of others. Somewhere in the middle are those who know they "should be" in therapy but who feel that their problems are not overwhelming and therefore believe they have ample time to deal with their issues. These individuals often act as if they must let the therapist know "something" that can be discussed but rarely let the therapist in very far, at least initially.

For those, like myself, who value self-disclosure and believe in its mutative influence, the task in working with individuals who are tentative about participating fully in therapy is to address this issue directly. "I have a sense that you're not sure what you really want to work on here." Or, even (if this is the case): "I'm not sure you believe you need to be here." Some patients may need explicit permission or encouragement to speak about less-than-urgent problems.

The Depth and Accessibility of the Problem

Some issues are intensely personal, close to the core of an individual's most fragile aspects of self (e.g., childhood abuse, sexual problems, family secrets), and therefore extremely painful to share with even a trusted other. Other problems, even those that cause moderate or severe distress (marital strife, bereavement), are often felt as less shameful and more discussable.

Of course, what is a deep core issue to one person may be far less so to another. The point, though, is that issues that make one feel fragile or personally vulnerable are going to be more difficult to discuss.

Somewhat related to depth is the issue of accessibility. What can a patient, even if strongly motivated, actually remember of highly charged events? On a very basic level, patients' disclosures are affected by what they can and can't remember and what has and has not been encoded verbally. Some patients never recollect the details of certain experiences, especially those that occurred in very early childhood. Often this is because early experiences are felt but not named; until named, they're not communicable through words. That is, the content of early experiences hasn't achieved the level of symbolization that makes verbal self-disclosure possible. Many object relations theorists (e.g., Winnicott) understood this well—that important preverbal events are basically ineffable. The therapist's task then is to try to find the words that match the patient's nonverbal and often unconscious attempts to communicate what has previously been uncommunicable.

The Nature of the Patient's Goals in Therapy

Some patients do not endorse understanding or insight as primary goals of therapy. They do not want to go deeply into their issues nor become more aware of the etiology or dynamics of their core conflicts. They do not believe that disclosure can be healing. They simply want to feel better (i.e., experience symptom relief) as soon as possible. They may want advice, and they may also want psychotropic medication, but they often do not want nor have the patience for those types of therapies that privilege disclosure as a means to therapeutic improvement.

But even patients who value disclosure may be circumspect in revealing their experiences. Some are eager to disclose as much as possible to their therapists, wanting to be known and understood fully; others want their therapists to know only about the particular problem(s) at hand. Thus, it is not unusual for some patients to be quite focal in their disclosures, omitting much about how they think, feel, and behave. To assess whether further work and greater disclosure is possible, I sometimes ask questions like: "Is there a part of you that would like to understand more about how or why this happened?" "Have you experienced any relief in having the opportunity to discuss this here in some detail?"

The Extent and Type of Patient Resistance

Resistance refers to the universal tendency to be withholding in therapy, to be not entirely open, present, or amenable to change. From a psychodynamic perspective, resistance reflects a patient's attempts to avoid painful feelings, especially shame, guilt, and loss. Resistance can be conceptualized as a more permanent character trait or as a temporary situation-specific state (Beutler, Moleiro, & Talebi, 2002). In the latter case, resistance may reflect a rupture in the therapeutic alliance. The patient may be resistant to disclose or explore with this particular therapist, in this particular setting, at this particular time.

Resistance is not, however, a pathological phenomenon but rather a normal process by which patients defend their sense of a stable self and strive to maintain their equilibrium when internal conflicts become too threatening or too close to the surface (Engle & Holiman, 2002). It may also be a means for patients to assert their healthy human need to be autonomous and separate from others, including the therapist (Messer, 2002). Some patients resist by avoiding emotionally charged topics; some by addressing critical issues but not getting any deeper into them as therapy progresses; some by chatting and flirtation; and some through blatant acting-out, for example, by coming late or missing appointments. Even a pattern of unconditional deferential agreement with the therapist may signal resistance—an attempt to avoid deep exploration of painful feelings through immediate superficial acquiescence.

There is a voluminous literature on dealing with patient resistance. Those writing about this topic consistently suggest that the first task is to understand the function of the resistance by engaging the patient in a discussion about this: "It feels to me that it's hard for you to open up here fully about your life. I'm wondering what your experience is of this." Until resistance is dealt with, honest and full patient disclosure about other important issues is unlikely.

The Nature of Patient Diagnosis and Character Type (Neurotic Style)

Patient diagnosis inevitably influences the nature and depth of self-disclosure. "A search for difficult truths about the self is possible for neurotic level people because their self-esteem is resilient enough to tolerate some unpleasant discoveries" (McWilliams, 1994, p. 69). On the other hand, patients who are psychopathic tend to withhold, distort, and lie as part of their typical symptom picture. Disclosure from these individuals, then, is unlikely to be entirely truthful. Similarly, patients who are narcissistic tend to present themselves in ways that suggest they are never responsible for their problems or issues; disclosure from this group is inevitably affected by their inability to see their own flaws.

A patient's neurotic style (Shapiro, 1999) also influences the nature and process of disclosure in therapy. For example, patients who are obsessional tend to focus on details when revealing, or concealing, their experiences. Clients with a more hysterical style tend to present information in a more diffuse and hard-to-pin-down manner. All this points to the need for therapists to be comprehensive in their assessments and to have a realistic awareness of how diagnosis and character style affect the disclosure process.

The Strength of the Therapeutic Relationship

The answer to many questions regarding what is effective about psychotherapy is "the relationship." A strong alliance, one marked by mutuality of tasks and goals, mutual regard, and likeability, has been consistently shown to be significantly associated with positive therapeutic outcome (Horvath & Bedi, 2002).

Many patients need to establish an effective therapeutic alliance before revealing their most difficult issues. Some will test their trust and faith in their therapists by working on less toxic issues in the beginning of therapy before they reveal the "hard stuff." Virtually all mental health professionals have had patients who have "hit them with a bombshell"—revealing, for example, a family secret, a history of abuse, a drug problem or a serious illness—well after therapy has begun. For the most part, these delayed revelations tend not to be of the kind where patients suddenly remember an earlier event (although this certainly occurs); rather, they are disclosures that are contingent upon the patient's perception of a necessary degree of safety.

Nevertheless, it is important to note that even a strong alliance, by itself, is no guarantee that critical aspects of a patient's inner world will necessarily emerge. As McWilliams (1994) has perspicaciously written: "I am not convinced that allowing a relationship to develop will create a climate of trust in which all pertinent material will eventually surface. Once the patient feels close to the therapist, it may become *harder* for him or her to bring up certain aspects of personal history or behavior" (p. 8). She offers the following example: "Most adults can answer questions about their sexual practices with relative frankness when talking to a professional who is still a stranger. But once the therapist has started to feel like a prudish mother or moralizing father, the words flow anything but easily" (pp. 15–16). Her point is that, once therapy has been well established, patients may experience a greater fear of rupturing an effective alliance or of derailing a movement toward self-acceptance. Relatedly, once a strong positive transference has developed, patients may be especially loath to speak about potentially shameful issues. However, my sense is that these phenomena are mitigated by patients' increasing trust in their therapists' acceptance of them. Furthermore, most therapists are aware of the importance of discussing the state of their relationship with their patients, especially emergent problems that may affect disclosure.

The Nature of the Therapeutic Contract

On a very basic level, the nature of the therapeutic contract—that is, whether therapy has been established as short-term and focused or long-term and open-ended—will directly affect the nature and extent of what is disclosed. The nature of short-term therapy virtually precludes in-depth exploration and disclosure of multiple issues. In fact, the short-term goals of rapid cognitive and behavioral change, in conjunction with an emphasis on confronting defenses, essentially precludes extensive accounts of the etiology of even targeted issues. On the other hand, the intense focus on defenses in short-term therapy may actually facilitate more rapid and deeper disclosures around a specific target issue than in longer-term open-ended therapies.

The Therapist's Attitudes toward and Responsiveness to Disclosures

A major influence on patient disclosure is rooted in a large constellation of "therapist factors," including the therapist's tendency to self-disclose (to be discussed at length in later chapters), the nature of his or her responses to patient disclosure (e.g., affirmation, silence, confrontation, attempts at clarification), and the extent to which he or she takes an active role in pursuing patient disclosures. Indeed, the results of a recent study by my research group (Farber, Berano, & Capobianco, 2004) suggest that many patients wish their therapists would more actively push them toward greater disclosure. It is also often the case that when therapists appear to be uncomfortable with certain disclosures (e.g., those that are abuse-related) patients either restrict further discussions of this topic or "sanitize" subsequent disclosures in the service of attenuating their therapist's discomfort. Therapists' own therapy and supervision are often indicated just for this reason: to make them more aware of how their responses (or blind spots) affect the process of therapy, including their patients' willingness to speak about difficult issues.

The Patient's Experience of Previous Disclosures

The appropriate cliché here is "Nothing succeeds like success." Patients who have experienced disclosures as difficult but worthwhile, who have come to trust their therapist to hear their deepest, most personal issues in a sensitive and accepting way, will naturally be more likely to continue exploring and disclosing private aspects of self. In this sense, self-disclosure is a recursive process. Conversely, those whose experiences with disclosure have been marked by shame, despair, or perceived insensitivity on the part of the listener are likely to resist opening up again. Of course, most patients in therapy have likely had both types of experiences as well as experiences wherein disclosures were concomitantly felt as satisfying and anxiety-provoking. Some patients need to talk about their previous experiences with disclosure, including their ambivalence and their perception of goodness of outcome, before they fully delve into new and seemingly difficult material.

LEGAL ISSUES, CONFIDENTIALITY, AND DISCLOSURE

Patient self-disclosure may be also affected by ethical and legal requirements. The current "Ethical Principles of Psychologists and Code of Conduct" of the American Psychological Association (2002) mandate that psychologists discuss the limits of confidentiality with those to whom they are providing services, specifying that "unless it is not feasible or is contraindicated, the discussion of confidentiality occurs at the outset of the relationship and thereafter as new circumstances may warrant" (p. 1066).

Although the information conveyed by a therapist about the specific limitations of confidentiality may ultimately apply to a small subset of therapy patients (i.e., those involved in forensic issues such as custody battles or other legal disputes; those who pose a danger to themselves or another; and those who are abusing children), no patient can be offered absolute confidentiality at the outset. The APA guidelines exist to ensure that patients understand the limits of confidentiality and are therefore equipped to make informed decisions about which personal information to disclose. Following the landmark Tarasoff case, in which a woman was killed by a patient who had voiced his homicidal ideation in therapy and whose therapist did not directly warn the potential victim, the Supreme Court significantly restricted the patient–therapist privilege in cases where there was reason to believe the patient might do harm to others: "The public policy favoring protection of the confidential character of the patient–psychotherapist communications must yield to the extent to which disclosure is essential to avert danger to others. The protective privilege ends where the public peril begins" (p. 24, *Tarasoff v. Board of Regents of the University of California*, 1976, as cited in Everstine et al., 1980). The boundaries of the therapeutic relationship were no longer inviolable—no longer exempt from the dictates of the courts or the needs of the larger society.

Bersoff (1976) was among the first to note that this case had profound implications for the conduct of psychotherapy: "Therapists may find themselves in insolvable conflicts as they attempt to reconcile their own personal morality and training regarding confidentiality, the vague reminders of their professional codes of ethics that warn of the consequences of violating the moral and legal standards of the community, and the developing legal requirements that demand complex decision making and a balancing between client and public interests" (p. 166). He also suggested that failure to convey these limits on confidentiality could ultimately result in a patient's loss of privacy and a therapist's loss of reputation.

Glosoff, Herlihy, Herlihy, and Spence, in their 1997 review of state laws related to privileged communication, noted an increasing number of exceptions to statutory psychologist–client privilege but also noted considerable variability in the strength and breadth of privilege afforded to the relationship. For example, with respect to the "duty to warn" exception that grew out of the *Tarasoff* case, states vary on such dimensions as whether the duty to warn extends to property as well as persons, whether the psychologist *must* or *may* warn, and to whom warnings should be given. Such variability led Glosoff et al. to recommend that psychologists stay current about their state's laws and court rulings, but also to go beyond the usual legal limits on disclosure and inform clients of the potential for court-ordered disclosure of information in other situations. Clients should be made aware, for example, that if they are thinking about introducing their emotional state into legal proceedings, some courts consider this an implied waiver of therapist–client privilege.

How does the legal establishment of limits to confidentiality affect patients' disclosure in therapy? Psychologists tend to believe that enumerating these limits has an inhibiting effect on disclosure—that as greater specificity is provided, the amount of information disclosed by patients becomes smaller (Haut & Muehleman, 1986). Nevertheless, research has not offered substantial support for this belief. In one study, Muehleman, Pickens, and Robinson (1985) found that providing potential clients (mildly depressed college students) detailed information regarding the limits to confidentiality was not generally detrimental to disclosure. Specifically, the results indicated that, although providing such information resulted in a decrease in one of seven categories ("mood"), even this effect was neutralized when a rationale for disclosure in therapy was provided in the consent form (i.e., stating that if the client was more open, the therapist would be better able to help him or her). The authors concluded that, if clinicians provide information about both the limits of confidentiality and the possible benefits of disclosure, "there will probably not be a significant inhibition of relevant self-disclosure in a therapeutic setting" (p. 395).

On the other hand, Kremer and Gesten (1998) found that providing information about managed care supervision and reporting requirements to clients resulted in significantly decreased self-disclosure. Unlike the participants in the Muehleman et al. (1985) study, clients in this study were not sufficiently convinced by the presentation of a persuasive rationale to maintain their willingness to disclosure.

In reflecting on these findings, it is important to remember that focusing on the average effect of patients' receipt of confidentiality information may cause us to overlook individual differences. For some patients (e.g., those who are currently involved in abusive or forensic situations), receiving explicit information about the limits of confidentiality may greatly influence disclosure, whereas for other patients such information is unlikely to have any effects. More generally, though, there may be significant differences in disclosure between those who are in "private" therapy and those involved in the managed care system—even when both groups are given the same information regarding the limits to confidentiality.

POSITIVE CONSEQUENCES OF SELF-DISCLOSURE IN PSYCHOTHERAPY

The nature and process of a patient's disclosures are influenced not only by those factors I've just described but also by the relative influence of the many positive and negative consequences of such behavior.

The positive aspects of all forms of interpersonal disclosure were described very briefly in the preceding chapter. Here, the discussion will focus on how they manifest specifically within the psychotherapeutic situation. What will be clear to most readers, though, is that the beneficial effects of disclosure per se cannot be differentiated from the more generally salutary effects of psychotherapy.

Intimacy

Disclosure is a means of forging or furthering a connection with another person; it is inherently relational (Skolnick & Messler Davies, 1992). In sharing intimate aspects of themselves, patients feel closer to their therapist. Even hurtful interpersonal disclosures may yield positive outcomes. It is not uncommon for a patient's expressed anger at his or her therapist to be met with acceptance in a way that forges a closer relationship.

Many therapists, especially those that adhere to a psychodynamic stance, set out rules of communication that call for intimacy and candor, attempting to limit what Kursh (1971) calls "pseudocommunicational events" in which only surface speech but no in-depth exploration of feelings occurs (p. 206). Still, this is a unique type of intimacy, one generally marked by a lack of true reciprocity in disclosure. Although the therapist inevitably discloses aspects of him- or herself through actions ranging from purposeful revelations of here-and-now feelings and personal information (e.g., vacation plans, number of children) to idiosyncratic speech patterns, choice of clothing, and office decorations, the focus in therapy is on the patient. It is the patient's needs that are primary, the patient's life that must be explored, and the patient's feelings, thoughts, and behaviors that must be discussed. On the one hand, then, patients do not learn nearly as much of the intimate details of their therapists' lives as vice versa (even as they do learn more than has traditionally been assumed); on the other hand, the depth and constancy of patient disclosures—even if mostly nonreciprocated—tend to create a sense of intimacy, especially when received in an empathic manner.

Moreover, patients' disclosures are often hard-fought, and the struggle to overcome shame amid the awareness of the therapist's availability and caring results typically in strong feelings of closeness in the dyad. Thus, as disclosure proceeds and the therapist learns more about the patient, and the patient learns more about the therapist, and they struggle together to make sense of this revealed material, a greater sense of intimacy develops in the relationship.

The development of intimacy through disclosure is illustrated by the following vignette.

> Julie, a 35-year-old divorced mother of two, had been in therapy with Dr. Samuel for nearly 2 years. Her presenting complaints included feelings of "sadness," "aloneness," "alienation from others," and "inability to form lasting relationships." Despite being urged for years by her family to attend therapy, this was her first such venture. During the first few months of therapy, Julie was tentative, self-deprecating, and on several occasions announced that she was not sure she was going to return for further sessions. In reporting her feelings or even her history—she was the older of two children raised by two very distant parents—she tended to speak in a monotonal fashion and punctuate her conversation with frequent observations that this "couldn't be of much interest" and that there was very little of her life that was special or noteworthy. But Dr. Samuel was an active and engaged listener, often querying Julie about specific details of her relationships with her parents or younger sister. In doing so, Julie began remembering more details of her childhood, including instances of parental fighting and drinking.
>
> Over time, Julie became increasingly involved in therapy, bringing in more material and doing so without questioning Dr. Samuel's interest in her. In fact, it became clear several months into the therapy that she began to look forward to her sessions. She would begin sessions with some newfound revelation—expounded upon with far greater affect than before—and would have trouble leaving at the end. Moreover, most of the sessions were marked by a good deal of give-and-take, of concerns or issues or memories supplied by Julie, of questions posed by Dr. Samuel, of thoughtful answers offered by Julie, of serious though occasionally playful observations made by Dr. Samuel.
>
> One could view the gradual improvement in Julie in terms of a transference cure, or in terms of the positive regard offered by Dr. Samuel, or in terms of cognitive restructuring ("I do have a more inter-

esting life and more positive attributes than I had thought")—and all are reasonable possibilities. But one means to all these outcomes was that Julie's disclosures resulted in a greater sense of intimacy. She felt she was in a relationship with her therapist. She felt cared for, in great measure a result of her increasingly greater willingness to disclose to her therapist.

Validation and Affirmation

As patients draw their therapist into their private worlds, enlisting help in understanding and changing their familiar though sometimes maladaptive ways of negotiating their lives, they may harbor certain wishes with regard to their therapist's response. Often, they seek reassurance, hoping that despite what they have thought or felt or done, the therapist will continue to think well of them and assure them that they are OK. (There are, of course, those cases where patients seem to do everything possible to get their therapists to dislike them, to accept their own view of themselves as unworthy of respect or care. Typically, however, work with these patients reveals their deep-seated hope for their therapist's care and approval.) When self-disclosure is met with the therapist's acceptance or reassurance, the patient feels validated. At that moment, he or she is both known and accepted—a powerful, self-enhancing feeling.

It is important to note, however, that the validation referred to here is not identical to that which Carl Rogers wrote about so eloquently. To Rogers, client validation emanates from the therapist's ability to be positively regarding and totally accepting of what he or she hears. In therapies that are more psychodynamically or even experientially based, validation may occur not just as a result of explicit affirmation or acceptance but also as a consequence of silence, challenge, or even confrontation. In his filmed work with Gloria (Shostrom, 1965)—the patient whose brief therapeutic sessions with Rogers, Perls, and Ellis served as the basis of what is probably the most often viewed video in training programs—Perls justifies his aggressive approach by remarking that it is because he respects her so much and insists on taking her seriously that he must call her on her "phoniness" and her attempts to hide from him like a "little girl." For some patients, a therapist's challenge—especially in response to a disclosure that seems superficial or misleading or one whose seemingly deep content is betrayed by a stylistic glibness—may represent the most affirming, validating response of all.

Kohut, the founder of self psychology, revolutionized psychoanalysis by his insistence on viewing narcissism as a healthy component of human development. All of us, he asserted (1971, 1977), have a great and innate need to find individuals in our environment who will affirm us, who will relate to us much the way that our ideal mothers served us during infancy. As fundamental as sex and aggression are, Kohut considered the need for self-esteem to be an equally potent force in understanding the dynamics of human development. According to this perspective, we disclose ourselves in order to get attention and approbation from others. Only when done excessively or obsessively does this very human tendency manifest as pathological narcissism.

Consistent with Kohut's views, the therapeutic value of being "known" by another has been one of the focal points of contemporary relational therapy. According to Jessica Benjamin (1988, 1992, 1998), true affirmation from the therapist is contingent upon the ability of the patient to recognize the therapist as a fully distinct other. Only by giving the therapist full recognition can the patient derive benefit from the therapist's recognition. From a metapsychological perspective, the patient's task is to move from seeing the therapist as "object" (a prototypical, nondistinct representation) to viewing him or her as "subject" (a distinct, individualized representation). The therapeutic goal, in Benjamin's paraphrase of Freud, is for patients to accomplish this transformation so that "where objects were, subjects must be" (1992, p. 44). In short, the therapeutic dyad provides the possibility for being both recognized and recognizing; from a relational perspective, one is impossible, and meaningless, without the other.

Mutual recognition may be seen as a developmentally higher achievement and one that adds a profound layer of meaning and satisfaction to the disclosure process. But, as the case below illustrates, it is surely not the means by which a therapist's affirmation can feel rewarding in the aftermath of patient disclosure.

> Beth was a 26-year-old public school teacher who had been sexually abused as a child by her father; she carried a diagnosis of borderline personality disorder with narcissistic features. Like many individuals who have been abused, her therapies—the current one was her fourth in the past 6 years—were marked by a lack of consistency. She would reveal a great amount of material about her experiences of being abused, then refuse to speak of these experiences at all; she would show up diligently and work hard in therapy, only to begin coming late and missing appointments. Beth would have great hopes for the therapy, feel that this therapist truly understood, and then would "crash" (her word) in the aftermath of an inevitable "misunderstanding." These ruptures would invariably center on their differences regarding Beth's culpability for the abuse. That is, she perceived her therapists' consistent attempts to exonerate her from her guilt ("what happened wasn't your fault; you were just a child") as well-meaning but misguided. From her perspective, these therapists simply did not hear her, did not take seriously her strong belief that she could have and should have done something more on her own behalf.

Her current therapy, with a student I supervise, has been somewhat more successful than her previous ones. Beth has been willing to stay longer in therapy and believes she is better able to tolerate the stresses of everyday living without frequent recourse to drugs, alcohol, or self-hatred. There are many reasons for this, but one part of the equation is that her therapist is able to provide affirmation for her in multiple ways. Beth's disclosures are agonizing, invariably replete with tears, rage, self-recrimination, and hopelessness. Her therapist is not only steadfast in her ability to listen well without judging but also manages to avoid the common beginner mistake of "making nice," that is, of disavowing too quickly or too reflexively a patient's sense of culpability in regard to awful experiences. Instead, this therapist has been able to affirm Beth through a combination of acknowledging the tragic elements in Beth's life while simultaneously praising her ability to face it: "It was awful, you did make some decisions you regret, you have paid a terrible price, and now you're managing to face all this shit. I admire your courage." The message that reached Beth was that despite her problems her therapist liked and respected her.

Insight and Identity Formation

A third benefit of patient disclosure lies in its potential to pull together previously fragmented aspects of a person's identity or, similarly, to strengthen those aspects that have felt diffuse or insubstantial. Through the process of selecting and narrating discrete aspects of self-experience, and through the therapist's emphasizing and clarifying those aspects that seem most prominent and enduring, patients may experience a more cohesive sense of self, successfully merging newly uncovered material with older, more familiar, self-representations. "I never realized that I was acting so similarly in these different situations." "I've come to be aware of the major themes in my life, my own ways of making sense of the world." In recent years, more therapists have become aware of the capacity of psychotherapy to increase an individual's "narrative coherence." In particular, the late Stephen Mitchell wrote extensively about the importance of this function of disclosure in psychotherapy. As Mitchell (2002) suggested, "We are our stories, our accounts of what happened to us . . . no stories, no self" (p. 145).

Using narrative to forge a more coherent identity is especially critical for patients who feel "all over the place," whose identity is fluid, whose sense of self is based too much on the needs and expectations of others. But virtually all patients in successful psychotherapy, especially those in dynamically oriented therapies, have been moved by their emerging awareness of the self's continuity, of how seemingly disparate events and experiences are related to a central theme or themes. Thus, as patients continue to disclose in therapy, they may well come to acknowledge a greater coherence in their sense of self.

> Bill, a 19-year-old college sophomore, was remarkably bright and psychologically sophisticated but also plagued by an inability to differentiate himself from his father, an extremely successful physician and generally strong-minded individual. Bill would vacillate between echoing his father's views (on everything from religion to politics) and repudiating everything his father stood for. The idea that he could forge an identity outside the realm of his father's beliefs was difficult to conceive. And, yet, he and his therapist managed to do just that. The therapist's gentle insistence on knowing what Bill thought and valued eventually allowed Bill to reveal much of his previously unacknowledged belief system, a good deal of which (not surprisingly) stood in opposition to his father's beliefs. In therapy, Bill was able to expose parts of himself that were frightening and/or unacceptable. He gradually became able to forge a sense of self that, while incorporating some elements of his father's values, essentially reflected his own emerging views of himself and the world.

Differentiation of Self

The converse of identity consolidation is identity differentiation: acknowledging and accepting disparate parts of oneself, especially feelings, behaviors, and thoughts that have previously been disavowed ("not me") or never allowed expression. Bromberg (1994) aptly terms this "the ability to stand in the spaces between realities without losing any, the capacity to feel like one self while being many" (p. 534). Thus, in the process of disclosing in psychotherapy, patients may become aware of roles or experiences that had not been part of their self-definition. Somewhat paradoxically, the greater the felt coherence in regard to one's identity, the greater the ability to discover and disclose multiple aspects of self.

Good therapists are often aware of what's left out of a patient's narrative or, more specifically, what aspects of self are not being expressed. They encourage patients to explore the conflict between contrasting self-images (e.g., positive and negative self-representations) and help patients accept the coexistence of multiple aspects of the self. Working with narratives that reveal how they may feel and act quite differently in different situations (see, for example, Bullitt & Farber, 2002), patients begin to accept the fact that they are more complex than they first realized and not bound to think of themselves in accordance with the expectations of others or their own narrow self-image.

Disclosure, then, has two complementary consequences: strengthening the coherence and stability of self-image, and increasing the complexity of the self-image by making patients aware of the multiplicity of their feeling states and behaviors. The process of disclosure in therapy, the gradual unfolding of self in the presence of another, enables patients to feel, paradoxically, both more unified and more differentiated.

> Stan, a 50-year-old man who had experienced abuse at the hands of his father, held but one consistent image of himself: as a survivor of abuse with serious impairments in the realm of interpersonal relationships. And while this was somewhat true, Stan did have a number of other attributes that he often failed to incorporate into his sense of self. He was a talented computer programmer, a knowledgeable fan of contemporary music, a good friend, and an avid reader. At the termination of a very long (9 years) and successful therapy that essentially ended with his ability to forge a committed relationship with a woman, we discussed some of what seemed to make a difference. "You were able to see parts of me that I couldn't see in myself, and you kept asking me about them. At first, I was annoyed, I just wanted to talk about the crap in my life, but at some point something changed. I began to like talking about how I was a good son and brother, and how I was a patient and sensitive listener to Rebecca. Eventually, these became parts of me."

Authenticity

Yet another consequence of sharing deeply personal aspects of self-experience is the patient's growing awareness of a greater sense of authenticity, of feeling more "real" and less fraudulent. As the space diminishes between what patients think or feel and what they say, they tend to feel far truer to themselves. At these moments they feel far more self-aware (having a heightened acceptance of deeper parts of themselves) than self-conscious (painfully experiencing shameful parts of themselves).

For most patients, monitoring and titrating disclosures to their therapists are stressful activities, interfering with their sense of personal integrity and image of an ideal self. Thus, the capacity to trust the therapist with personal information tends to be emotionally freeing and a source of pride. Sharing intimate feelings rather than just thoughts or behaviors is an especially effective means for experiencing authenticity—and this may be even more the case when strong positive or negative feelings about the therapist are disclosed.

> Laura is a 45-year-old woman who has suffered from dysthymia for many years. The focus of her life is her work as a civil servant. She has had few intimate relationships in her life with either men or women. She is likable and smart but is keenly aware of always feeling one step

removed from others and one step removed from her own feelings. She describes them as existing outside of her. When I don't encourage Laura to speak of her feelings—toward me, toward friends in her life, toward coworkers—she is often content to relate the work-connected events of the week, filling me in on "what's new." But when I do get her to talk about her feelings, including rage toward her absent father, jealousy toward her favored brother, resentment toward her better-paid colleagues, and feelings of emotional closeness with and sexual attraction toward me—her schizoid core begins to give way and her demeanor shifts dramatically. She is there, fully in the room, aware of many of the feelings that she reflexively avoids out of discomfort and shame. She recognizes the difference between these two ways of being. For the most part, she enjoys feeling more alive and is working hard to embrace this kind of authenticity in her life outside of therapy.

Catharsis

Lastly, and many would say most importantly, patients benefit from sharing private material with their therapist by experiencing relief from the often overwhelming burden of keeping painful memories, thoughts, and feelings to themselves. In one of Yalom's novels, the protagonist (a fictionalized Nietzsche) says: "It seems to me that the more I am able to tell of my innermost feelings, the more relief I will gain" (1992, p. 159). As patients reveal information that has been either unconsciously repressed or consciously suppressed, they may sigh, sweat, stutter, hyperventilate, shake their heads, and cry. Indeed, our idioms suggest that we harbor emotions in our bodies until they are disclosed: We need to "get things off our chest," "get it out of our system," or "blow off steam" (Smyth, 1998).

Research has shown that keeping secrets is often accompanied by significant physiological and psychological symptomatology. Larson and Chastain (1990) found that high self-concealers report more depression, anxiety, and physical symptoms than do low self-concealers. And Wegner and Lane (1995) found that active suppression tends to lead to intrusive thoughts about the very things that people are trying to suppress. According to their "preoccupation model of secrecy," these thoughts may become the bases for psychopathology. For example, bereaved mothers who were discouraged or barred from disclosing their experience manifested higher levels of intrusive thoughts and depressive symptomatology (Lepore, Silver, Wortman, & Wayment, 1996).

Bass and Davis (1988) understood the power of catharsis in encouraging survivors of abuse to tell their stories: "It helps to name your fears. Naming things gives them less of a hold" (p. 185). But there is something else that occurs as a consequence of self-disclosures that their example doesn't quite capture. This act, at its most powerful, not only serves to discharge toxic emotions but also serves a redemptive function. Like confession in its most spiritual sense, disclosure brings a state of grace, of absolution. I have not just let go of what is toxic and therefore feel free of dysphoric feelings; I have also created a strongly positive self-state. Disclosure then may not just engender a state of peacefulness but may produce new feelings of wholeness and virtue.

> Amanda is 34, a mother of three, a wife in an emotionally distant relationship. She suffers from posttraumatic stress disorder (PTSD), the result of being sexually abused by her grandfather when she was a young adolescent. She repressed knowledge of these events until a required college paper flooded her with vivid memories, images, and shame. She now has recurrent nightmares, startle responses, and is, in general, emotionally labile. She "detests" talking about what happened to her all those years ago and does so only when the nightmares increase in intensity or when intrusive thoughts interfere with her ability to be an effective mother. At these times, she relates graphically what occurred and is able to express (often through the use of obscenities) her feelings toward the perpetrator as well as toward those family members, especially her own mother, who did nothing to prevent the abuse, despite knowing that this man had been sexually abusive to others before. These sessions provide an outlet for expressing intense and difficult feelings. They allow Amanda to vent and rage and cry. They serve to absolve her from assuming an unwarranted sense of responsibility for what occurred. These disclosures also move Amanda to regard herself as more worthy in God's eyes, as more deserving of His grace. And, finally, they enable her to get on with the other tasks of life, like motherhood, that she regards as sacred.

NEGATIVE ASPECTS OF DISCLOSURE IN PSYCHOTHERAPY

Based solely on this list of potentially positive consequences of disclosure, one might conclude that this is a no-lose situation. Patients disclose and feel better; they disclose and even therapists feel better (i.e., helpful and involved). Nevertheless, as all therapists know, even individuals whose primary experience is one of relief at having revealed something difficult may concomitantly experience dysphoric feelings. As one of my patients astutely commented, "I hate the fact that I have to work so hard here in order to feel ashamed."

The following represent the most salient negative aspects of patient disclosure, corresponding in large measure to the list of dysfunctional consequences of interpersonal disclosures noted briefly in the preceding chapter. The fact that patients will inevitably experience at least some of these effects underscores the complexity of disclosure in therapy and the need for an exquisite degree of sensitivity on the part of therapists.

Fear of Rejection

"You're going to hate me if I tell you what I did. You're not going to want me as your patient anymore." When shame is externalized and projected onto the therapist, it often appears as fear of rejection. Moreover, because most self-disclosures include a subtle or not-so-subtle wish for approval, patients may experience their therapist's questioning or even neutrality as devastating. "Oh, my God, why is he asking so many questions? He should just be comforting me." Or: "Why is she saying that? It seems like she's actually taking my husband's side." Thus, like all interpersonal disclosures, patient disclosures are fraught with the fear that the listener will be judgmental or critical. Some patients, then, are apprehensive that their disclosures may give their therapists "ammunition" with which to hurt or reject them. Disclosures reflecting a patient's feelings toward his or her therapist—feelings of disappointment, closeness, anger, or any other intense interpersonal experience—are especially likely to be accompanied by apprehension over the therapist's reaction.

Related to the fear or actuality of rejection following a disclosure is the fear of being taken advantage of. This is most often seen in a patient's reluctance to disclose improved financial circumstances for fear that the therapist will raise his or her fee.

Fear of Burdening the Therapist

Patients may feel anxious or even angry if they perceive that their therapist is reluctant to hear traumatic material because he or she may also have "been there" (e.g., experienced divorce, parental death, or serious illness). Furthermore, if the patient's fears are at all realized—if the therapist does become judgmental or nonplussed by certain disclosures—therapeutic progress is likely to be impaired. Similarly, patients may feel that they have to protect their therapist from some disclosures, especially if they perceive their therapist as too young or inexperienced to handle raw (e.g., intensely sexual or aggressive) material. Of course, sometimes this fear is more in the service of protecting the self than of the therapist.

As noted earlier in this chapter, some patient disclosures may, in fact, be difficult for the therapist to hear, especially when he or she has suffered from similar experiences. These disclosures may revive aspects of the therapist's most painful moments and most difficult relationships. This is why some therapists seem to collude with a patient's reluctance to speak of these issues. While in the short run patients may feel relieved that their therapist has not actively pursued this information, those who sense that they are protecting their therapists from difficult-to-hear material will inevitably resent the limitations of their relationship.

Fear of Creating Undesirable Impressions of Oneself

Closely connected to the preceding two scenarios is the fear that the more undesirable aspects of self that are being explored in therapy will become the primary basis of the therapist's judgments and attitudes. A supervisee of mine once reported a patient saying the following to her: "I'm afraid that you [my therapist] will think of me as more depressed and pathological than I am because that's all we talk about." In fact, Kelly's (2000) research led her to conclude that patients may be better off not disclosing shameful details of their lives because they risk losing their therapist's positive appraisal of them. Most clinicians and researchers reject this notion, averring that competent, well-trained therapists treat their patients' disclosures in a sensitive, nonjudgmental manner and continue to exhibit respect in the face of virtually all "disreputable" revelations. Nevertheless, some patients, especially those with acute interpersonal fears (e.g., those with personality disorders) may believe otherwise and become quite anxious in the aftermath of disclosing difficult material.

Conversely, there may be a fear that certain disclosures will alter one's self-perception. A patient of mine feared disclosing the details of her mom's hurtful behavior toward her because in doing so she would no longer be "mommy's good girl." Another had intense difficulty in coping with the changes in her self-image wrought by disclosures of her sexual excitement when she was abused. Yet another patient who disclosed extensively about her experiences of being abused struggled to avoid seeing herself exclusively in terms of "abuse victim." The point is that, as psychotherapy encourages openness about uncomfortable or troubling aspects of the self, these disturbing facets may come to dominate one's self-image. As novelist John Irving noted, "You can become tyrannized by the authenticity of what you remember" (cited in Gussow, 1998, p. E1).

Regret for Hiding So Long

Patients may feel ashamed, even pathetic, over the fact that they have been pretending or hiding from self and others for so long. "I feel so stupid at having kept this to myself all these years. It feels so childish." There is a sense here of waste, of wasted years and wasted opportunities. Thus, while the process of revealing previously hidden material may feel liberating and rejuvenating, these feelings may co-occur with a good deal of self-deprecation for having avoided this disclosure until now.

Feelings of Increased Vulnerability

Patients may feel that intimate disclosures of shameful material deprive them of a safe protective space. Especially acute is the apprehension, or actual experience, of being overwhelmed by what has been disclosed—the sense that old and painful memories are flooding the stream of consciousness, that feelings are spilling over, and that it may be impossible "to keep it all together." Some worry that deep disclosures will lead to irreversible pain and vulnerability. Others fear that further digging and disclosing will bring them uncomfortably close to "forbidden knowledge," perhaps something related to parental sexual activity.

In a related vein, some self-disclosures virtually preclude the continued repetition of secretive but typically pleasurable behavior. As one patient admitted to me, "If I tell you my secret, I may have to stop doing what I'm doing." Those who reveal their guilty pleasures (e.g., illicit sex, gambling, substance abuse, criminal activity, or reckless driving) often desperately want such behaviors to cease and may even want their therapist's help in effecting these changes. Still, they have typically kept this activity private as a result of their unwillingness to give up this seemingly vital part of their lives—and may feel quite vulnerable without it. Some patients also fear that their therapist may respond to a disclosure with advice they may not want to hear (e.g., "If you're so unhappy, why not consider divorce?"). More generally, the events or feelings disclosed may shatter long-held patterns of effective functioning, including the effective use of defenses. "I've managed to deal with this issue, managed to keep it under wraps for so long—why did I bother to unwrap it now?"

Feelings of Shame

To briefly reiterate what has already been emphasized: Shame is a frequent concomitant of disclosure in psychotherapy (Broucek, 1991; Livingston & Farber, 1996; Wurmser, 1981), affecting the timing, focus, and depth of what is discussed. Patients often experience shame or guilt following the disclosure of a deeply held secret; they may then have to cope with intense self-loathing images. "I can't believe I did that; I hate that piece of myself." They tend to feel exposed and powerless in the presence of the therapist to whom they have just opened up. They may want to run from therapy to escape these feelings. "It's so hard for me to have you know this about me. I feel like a stupid little kid."

However, feelings of shame are not at all confined to confessions of past transgressions. In fact, sometimes the most shameful (and vulnerable) moments in therapy are when patients acknowledge intense feelings of dependency on or love for their therapist, especially when such feelings are accompanied by romantic or erotic fantasies.

DISCLOSURE IN THERAPY: THE CASE OF THE ABUSED PATIENT

Conflicts surrounding disclosure may be especially acute for abused patients for whom shame is such a central aspect of experience. Furthermore, their concerns about trust, vulnerability, and their basic capacity for human relatedness often give their disclosures a different feeling, almost as if they serve different purposes and operate under a different set of contingencies than what has been outlined so far.

In particular, I am thinking of those abused individuals for whom self-disclosure is a means not so much to further understand thoughts and feelings, or even to achieve a state of relief from emotional pain, as it is to elicit certain emotional responses from their therapist. These patients, who have often experienced states of depersonalization and alienation, may selectively disclose those events or feelings they perceive will evoke their therapists' compassion and recognition, responses that make them feel more part of the world and worthy of care. Or, they may invent or exaggerate disclosures in order to gain approval from their therapists. Goffman (1959) used the metaphor of theatrical performance to describe the process by which we all attempt to guide and control the impressions others form of us through our behavior. All patients seek their therapist's approval, but patients who have been abused or otherwise traumatized may be desperate for such approbation. Since a lack of approval may be experienced as psychological annihilation for such patients, approval becomes perceived as a virtual life-or-death matter. Patients may thus weave elaborate narratives of success, including therapeutic success, that far exceed reality.

Similarly, survivors of abuse may distort or invent experiences in an attempt to force intimacy. These lies may not serve the same purposes that "normal" lies sometimes serve, such as avoiding difficulties or escaping punishment or censure. Instead, these false disclosures (e.g., exaggerated similarities between themselves and their therapists) are often desperate attempts to foster a sorely lacking sense of closeness or belonging. As one survivor bluntly describes it; "I lied all the time. I didn't tell lies to get out of trouble. I told them to erase differences. . . . I'd lie so I could make connections with people" (quoted in Bass & Davis, 1988, p. 388). In the process, these survivors succeed in accomplishing the opposite of what they had set out to do: instead of making themselves known to another, they obscure their true self beneath lies and masks. Thus, the core of their trauma festers untouched and leads typically to further alienation. Not only is intimacy hindered in the present, but also the mutative power of future disclosures may be compromised. In fact, if or when the need for true sharing becomes pressing, these survivors may have enormous difficulties in expressing what was hidden and distorted for so long.

Feelings of estrangement or depersonalization may also lead patients to disclose in order to prove to their therapist and themselves that they possess authentic "human" feelings. An adult survivor of childhood sexual abuse (CSA) poignantly relates how and why this might occur: "The ironic thing is, I tell people incredibly intimate things very quickly. It's an appearance of intimacy. I'd hear myself saying these 'really honest things.' But I said them so many times that they were just blunt instruments. The other person would react like I was taking them into my confidence, but I knew it was all fake. . . . It was just an appearance of belonging to the human race" (quoted in Bass & Davis, 1988, p. 388).

Finally, disclosure among patients who have been abused may achieve a certain paradoxical quality. That is, as a consequence of reporting positively tinged memories or feelings, certain patients experience distress. Why? Because these patients often have strong needs to maintain a harsh negative identity that has become familiar and feels authentic. Furthermore, since these patients fear that too much improvement will lead a therapist to conclude they no longer need therapy, persistently self-disparaging narratives guard against fears of abandonment. Patients who have survived abuse often need to manipulate the image they present to the therapist so that it remains within the bounds of neediness, though not excessive neediness that might push the therapist away. Sometimes these overwhelming, often contradictory, elements of disclosure lead to a verbal "stuckness" in abused patients that manifests in somaticized forms of communication to therapists (e.g., coughing, leg pains, or breathing difficulties).

DEALING WITH DISCLOSURE: WHAT DO PATIENTS AND THERAPISTS DO?

Disclosure brings with it so many potential conflicts. What do patients do? In practice, patient disclosures may be impulsive, guided by momentary fears, anxieties, or needs rather than by a cohesive long-term strategy. Still, there may be characteristic patterns. For example, there are those patients who, fearful of the potential dysfunctional effects of disclosure (perhaps because they've already had such experiences), essentially opt out of the process. These are the individuals who adopt the maxim "Let sleeping dogs lie." Some even seem to adhere to the tenet "Let rabid dogs lie." In either case, such individuals may seek psychotherapy for symptom relief but cling to the belief that "shit happens" and there's no use in talking much about it. I mentioned such patients earlier in a discussion of how patients' goals affect the process of disclosure in therapy. These are the patients who call to mind a *New Yorker* cartoon in which a patient says to his therapist: "Look, call it denial if you like, but I think what goes on in my personal life is none of my own damn business."

On the other end of the continuum are those patients who seem to have little or no difficulty in disclosing nearly everything of importance, from painful aspects of their past to intense here-and-now feelings toward their therapist.

For most patients, though, both sides of the disclosure equation tend to play out. That is, they divulge intimate information to their therapists and suffer both distress and relief in doing so, the proportions of which vary as a consequence of the type and timing of the disclosure, as well as how it is received. Moreover, disclosure and concealment invariably co-occur: Even as patients are disclosing they are also concealing; even as they are concealing, they are disclosing something of themselves. Thus, it is important for therapists to keep in mind that patient disclosure and concealment are in dialectical opposition to each other—seemingly opposite but, in fact, complementary. The existence of each is constant even though the balance between them is constantly changing.

In addition, depending on the disclosure and the way it is received, distress may linger and relief (e.g., resolution of pain) may not be experienced immediately after the disclosure. Thus, in the moment, there may be concomitant feelings of wanting to reveal more and regretting having spoken at all, a conflict well described by the phrase in REM's song "Losing My Religion," that goes "Oh no I've said too much / I haven't said enough."

Ambivalence can also be observed in disclosures that occur at the very end of sessions, sometimes even as patients are walking out the door. These "parenthetic," "by-the-way" statements are often extremely meaningful, but because they happen with little or no time left in the session, they may go unremarked upon by the therapist at the time. Many therapists do note that "this will have to be discussed next time," and many will speak at the next session about the process issues involved, that is, wondering aloud why the patient felt compelled to introduce such an important issue with no time left in the session for discussion. The usual reason, of course, again lies in the conflicted attitude of patients in regard to highly charged disclosures. Thus, a compromise solution is sought, one in which patients attempt to feel safe and somewhat hidden, even as they disclose something of great importance.

Importantly, however, for those who remain in therapy the more positive, healing aspects of disclosure tend to predominate. In fact, recent research (Farber et al., 2004) points strongly to a temporal model wherein patients' initial apprehension regarding disclosure and their sense of vulnerability during disclosure yield over time to feelings of relief, authenticity, safety, and pride. It is as if before disclosure patients feel more fragile than otherwise, and after disclosure they feel more resilient than otherwise. The results of this study also indicate that most patients tend not to regret disclosures and, indeed, believe that intimate disclosures in therapy facilitate subsequent disclosures to their therapist as well as to other significant individuals in their life.

What's a therapist to do with patients' oft-conflicted feelings around disclosure? Some, like the therapist depicted in Wise's (2004) poignant account of her own long-term treatment, believe in pushing for increasingly more intimate disclosures: "What haven't you told me?" (p. 64). Or, similarly:

> "What don't you want to talk about?"
> "My childhood."
> "Okay, let's start there." (p. 66)

For this severely depressed patient, this approach worked well: "I found myself hoping that she could find the way for me to talk more openly to her about my feelings" (p. 49). It helped, of course, that this therapist was not just confrontational (as these examples might imply) but also exquisitely sensitive, patient, genuine, and positively regarding. Another tack is to ask the patient directly whether there are things left unsaid about the topics under discussion. I like the simple elegance in Ornstein's (2005) question: "Is there anything more you are struggling to say or not to say about this?" (p. 113). Still other therapists attempt to increase the domain of "allowable" disclosures—in essence, educating the patient that all sorts of things may be usefully discussed in therapy, from events of the past to current feelings about the therapist to seemingly strange beliefs or experiences.

By contrast, other therapists believe strongly in allowing the patient to reveal at his or her own speed and discretion. In practice, this stance may mean that some issues, even those that the therapist believes might be profitably addressed, may never be. The dilemma over how far to push a patient to reveal intimate material, including his or her feelings toward the therapist, is a central aspect of one of the more difficult challenges in psychotherapy: when to respect a patient's defenses and when to confront them.

The therapist who remains keenly aware of the potential positive and negative consequences of patient disclosure—and perhaps especially aware of a patient's favored position on the expression–repression continuum—is likely to react appropriately to the presence or absence of revelations that occur in sessions. Most often, this involves responding to disclosures with empathy and acceptance. Still, as noted earlier, other responses are sometimes indicated, including silence, gentle questioning, and mutual exploration of the disclosure process. These responses may be especially indicated when the patient has offered some hint, verbal or otherwise, that he or she does want certain material pursued but finds it difficult to do so. Sometimes, too, therapist disclosure may be a helpful response to (or precipitant of) patient disclosures, one that may reinforce or deepen such disclosures and strengthen the therapeutic relationship. Conversely, an inappropriate, clumsy, or poorly timed response on the part of the therapist is likely to compromise therapeutic closeness, causing at least temporary ruptures in the alliance. The therapist's attitude, words, and tone are all likely to significantly affect the depth, ease, and pace of a patient's disclosures.

Virtually every patient is faced with two related dilemmas during every therapy session: "What should I discuss today?" and "Whatever I discuss, how completely honest and open should I and can I be?" These decisions are influenced, virtually on a moment-to-moment basis, by the therapeutic interaction. Indeed, at different times, for different issues, at different points in the discussion, different patients need different things from their therapists, including sometimes "permission" to stop or even not to disclose. In fact, many patients have an intuitive sense of how far they have usefully gone in their exploration of a particular issue, at least at this particular time in their therapy. Despite my general sense that disclosure is an integral aspect of therapy, a patient's reluctance to go any further—especially after being encouraged to do so—is likely to represent a degree of wisdom that therapists need to respect.

Finally, it is worth reiterating that, although patient disclosure is most often facilitated by "gentle" therapist responses (e.g., empathy), contrary means of fostering this process are possible. Perls' aggressive treatment of Gloria is one example. But here I have in mind an anecdote related by a good friend of mine, a therapist himself. In thinking about choosing a new therapist many years ago, he remained aware of his own tendency—so true of so many of us in the field—to use his considerable intellect to charm, hide, avoid, and distance himself from therapists and the stuff that most needed to be addressed. With this in mind, with the notion that he wanted someone who would not let him get away with his "usual shit," he chose "the most confrontational, biggest son of a bitch" he had encountered as a supervisor to be his therapist. Years later, he reports that it was a difficult but highly successful therapy.

CHAPTER 3

Research Perspectives on Patient Disclosure

Finally, never forget that you have promised to be absolutely honest, and never leave anything out because, for some reason or other, it is unpleasant to tell it.
—FREUD (1913, p. 135)

The first lesson of my life: Nobody can face the world with his eyes open all the time.
—RUSHDIE (1991, p. 142)

Freud's (1913) "fundamental rule," that the patient must disclose every thought that comes to mind, is almost certainly unfeasible. Few, if any, individuals can or will allow themselves the freedom to express themselves that completely. Because patients struggle with unexpurgated disclosure in therapy, and because the healing process is inextricably related to the material that is made available within the therapeutic relationship, researchers have begun to investigate the types, extent, process, and effects of patient disclosure. This chapter summarizes the empirical work on these and related issues.

"There are things I could never tell you," a patient of mine once remarked. "It would absolutely overwhelm me to go there." "What do you suppose would happen," I asked, "if you ever did tell me these things?" "I'd just disintegrate, I'd fall apart, I'd never come back." For this patient, the events in question were incidents of brutal childhood sexual and physical abuse, events that in large measure she felt responsible for eliciting.

However, the range of taboo topics, of issues that are difficult or seemingly impossible to discuss even in therapy, is both infinitely broad and idiosyncratic. What is woefully difficult for one patient to discuss may be surprisingly easy for another. Nevertheless, a smattering of such topics may be gleaned from popular movies and stories that have frequently used psychotherapy as a thematic frame. In Hitchcock's classic movie *Spellbound*, the protagonist (Gregory Peck) literally swoons when pushed by his therapist/lover (Ingrid Bergman) to remember a murder he witnessed, one that reminded him of a tragic childhood accident in which he was involved. In Peter Shaffer's powerful play *Equus*, the adolescent protagonist (Peter Firth) sings popular commercial jingles during therapy as a means of avoiding memories of shameful sexual experiences and his own cruelty to the horses that observed him. In both the book and movie *The Prince of Tides*, memories of being raped and killing the perpetrators are nearly impossible to access from the repressed memory of the central character and only become available as a result of the therapist's unethical seduction. In *Good Will Hunting*, the brilliant, angry young adult (Matt Damon) resists engagement with multiple therapists, and it is only the unconventional therapist (Robin Williams) to whom he reluctantly confides his secret of being physically abused as a child. In the underrated novel *August* (by Judith Rossner), the client in a long-term psychoanalytic therapy feels blocked trying to remember early experiences of being abandoned by her parents. And, in the wonderful book (by Judith Guest) and equally compelling movie (directed by Robert Redford) *Ordinary People*, the protagonist (Timothy Hutton) struggles mightily to acknowledge to his therapist (Judd Hirsch) his feelings about his brother's tragic death, including sadness, anger, and survivor guilt.

Deeply traumatic issues not only are the stuff of Hollywood movies but also constitute much of the work of long-term therapy. Despite managed care's pressure to focus on short-term symptom reduction, many clinicians, especially those practicing within a psychodynamic framework, continue to work with patients for month and years on long-standing characterological issues. The assumption of these therapists, one shared by many of their patients, is that awareness of deep-rooted psychological issues is of profound value even in the absence of immediate or extensive symptomatic relief, adding immeasurably to self-knowledge and the ability to live life more fully. Thus, although many in the psychological community have lessened their once unshakable faith in the curative power of insight and awareness (e.g., Wheelis, 1958), many others still adhere to the belief that greater awareness of self, achieved in great measure through accessing early memories and disclosing and analyzing current and past experiences, is of enormous import. From a less psychodynamic and more straightforward perspective, "the more open and revealing clients are about their thoughts and feelings, the more therapists ought to be able to help them" (Hill, Thompson, Cogar, & Denman, 1993, p. 278).

THE EXTENT OF PATIENT DISCLOSURE
AND NONDISCLOSURE

The freedom to disclose one's most private experiences is ensured by the knowledge that, with few exceptions, whatever is shared in therapy will be held in the strictest confidence by the person to whom it is disclosed. Sometimes this sense of safety is sufficient for patients to talk freely; sometimes, even within this very private and confidential space, patients are unable to overcome fears and doubts and so remain relatively hidden. As noted in the preceding chapter, most patients strive to find a comfortable place along a continuum of "safe disclosure," at times feeling they have disclosed too much (with resultant feelings of shame and vulnerability), at other times feeling too closed and defensive (with resultant feelings of frustration, wasted time, and/or self-abasement).

Research on patient disclosure in therapy—on what types of thoughts and feelings are and are not discussed and the reasons underlying nondisclosure—is surprisingly scant. Some of Jourard's (1971a, 1971b) early research included the "therapist" as a potential disclosure recipient, but the subjects in these analogue-type studies were not patients but rather college students asked to imagine which topics they would or would not disclose to a therapist. Yalom (1970) and Norton, Feldman, and Tafoya (1974) found that participants in encounter groups were most likely to withhold sexual secrets and feelings of either inadequacy or alienation.

Among the first group of researchers to systematically investigate disclosure in individual therapy, Hill and her colleagues (Hill et al., 1992, 1993; Regan & Hill, 1992; Thompson & Hill, 1991) proposed three separate, though overlapping, categories of client "covert processes": hidden reactions, things left unsaid, and secrets. Hidden reactions refer to "thoughts and feelings clients have in response to specific therapist interventions" (p. 278). Things left unsaid "refer to thoughts or feelings clients have during sessions that they do not share with their therapist" (p. 278); these are not necessarily in reaction to specific therapist interventions. Secrets "are major life experiences, facts, or feelings that clients do not tell their therapists" (p. 278). These three phenomena, although differing along the dimension of immediacy of nondisclosure (i.e., for how long the client has withheld significant information), all represent ways of keeping thoughts and feelings private, out of a therapist's awareness. Arguably, a fourth category of concealment, yet to be empirically studied, is client distortion or outright dishonesty, either through lying (inventing events that did not happen) or through the deliberate twisting of actual events. This may be an especially common occurrence among those patients suffering from drug or alcohol abuse, those with a diagnosis of antisocial personal disorder, and those involved in complicated legal actions (Newman & Strauss, 2003).

Several of Hill's studies (Hill et al., 1992, 1993; Thompson & Hill, 1991) have found that clients hide immediately experienced negative reactions (e.g., feeling scared, confused, misunderstood, or stuck) more often than they hide positive reactions (e.g., feeling understood, supported, or hopeful). These findings are consistent with Rennie's (1992, 1994) earlier work indicating that clients in therapy often operate at two parallel levels simultaneously: a level that features cooperation and pleasantness and a concomitant level of resentment and doubt. The participants in Rennie's studies admitted being reluctant to express negative feelings, with many averring either that it was not "their place" to challenge their therapist's expertise, that it was somehow petty or unfair to raise criticisms of their therapist in the context of a therapy that was essentially helpful, or that such criticism might jeopardize an otherwise good relationship. In short, the findings of Hill and Rennie suggest that many clients have bought into the idea that "If you can't say something nice, don't say it at all." Consequently, therapists sometimes have to actively encourage patient disclosure of negative feelings. As one therapist expressed it, "Somehow, I have to help you tell me" (Wise, 2004, p. 96).

How often do clients hold back information from their therapist? Almost two-thirds of the long-term clients in Hill et al.'s (1993) study acknowledged leaving something unsaid during sessions (thoughts or feelings not shared with their therapist) and almost half admitting having secrets, most either sexual in nature or related to feelings of failure. In Kelly's (1998) study, 40.5% of clients acknowledged that they were keeping a "relevant" secret from their therapist; most often, these secrets reflected either relationship difficulties or sexual issues. And, in an early study of "what patients don't tell their therapists," Weiner and Shuman (1984) found that 42% of their subjects had withheld information from their therapists. In Pope and Tabachnick's (1994) study, only 20% of the participants admitted that there was something "important they had kept secret and refused to disclose to any therapist" (p. 251); by far, the most widely noted category was "sexual issues." However, this was a sample of psychologists, a group that we would expect to exhibit lower rates of nondisclosure to their own therapists. In sum, it does appear that a substantial proportion of therapy patients, perhaps between 40 and 50% among nontherapists, keep secrets in therapy, most of which are reflective of long-term relational and sexual concerns.

However, if we narrow the domain and focus only on concealment of process issues (what occurs in the here and now between the participants in the room), we'd derive numbers that would seem to suggest that clients hide very little in therapy. For example, in Hill et al.'s (1992) study, only 14% of all client reactions were hidden, and in other studies conducted by Hill's research team (Hill et al., 1993; Regan & Hill, 1992) clients were found, on average, to report only one thing they failed to say to their therapist in a given session. It is also noteworthy that therapists in the Hill et al.

(1993) study were seldom aware of what their clients withheld in therapy. That is, despite clinical lore (dating from Freud) that patients inevitably "betray" their secrets through slips of the tongue or observable body language, they usually do not. Patients can and do conceal information from their therapist, often quite readily and easily.

Choosing an appropriate methodology to investigate either long-term secrets or nondisclosure of immediately experienced feelings or thoughts is difficult. As has been consistently noted, clients often refrain from disclosing fully to their therapist out of fear or shame, and these same processes are likely to be operative in responding to researchers as well. Furthermore, open-ended questions that focus on client secrets (e.g., "What, if any, thoughts or feelings did you have during the session that you did not share with your therapist?") render disclosure an "either–or" proposition rather than a phenomenon that may vary along a continuum, ranging from no disclosure whatsoever (that is, a total secret) to partial disclosure to extensive disclosure. In "real life," most patients are neither fully disclosing nor fully secretive but rather somewhere in between for virtually all their most intimate issues, a fact not taken into account by most current methodologies. To remedy this problem, my colleagues and I have been assessing the extent to which clients disclose a wide range of topics to their therapists in a series of studies over the past decade (Farber, 2003; Farber et al., 2004; Farber & Hall, 2002; Farber & Sohn, 1997, 2001; Hall & Farber, 2001; Pattee & Farber, 2004; Roe & Farber, 2001).

WHAT ISSUES ARE DISCUSSED MOST EXTENSIVELY IN PSYCHOTHERAPY?

For the first of our studies (Farber & Hall, 2002; Hall & Farber, 2001), we recruited 147 psychotherapy patients, most of whom were white, female, in their mid-thirties, well educated, and in long-term treatment with therapists practicing from a psychodynamic or eclectic orientation.

We asked them to fill out the Disclosure-to-Therapist Inventory—Revised (DTI-R), a questionnaire developed specifically to assess the extent of patients' disclosure on a wide range of intimate topics in therapy. Before discussing what we found, let's return for a moment to the methodological question raised a few paragraphs ago, essentially: "If patients aren't willing to disclose to their therapists about these issues, why would they disclose to you?" Several answers arise in response to this intriguing question (invariably the question that gets asked first at professional conferences). First, there's the "stranger on the train" phenomenon—the tendency for individuals to share secrets with those whom they believe they will never see or hear from again. Patients may feel less vulnerable speaking with researchers than with their therapist because the former relationship is less intimate. Second, and relatedly, despite the shameful aspects of secrets, there's also nearly universal pressure to share them with someone—often in the service of either confession ("I did something terrible that I've never told anyone about before") or self-aggrandizement ("I once did this wild, amazing thing that I haven't told anyone about in 20 years"). And third, the paradigm employed in these studies doesn't include requests for the details of secrets. Instead, patients are asked to rate the extent of their disclosure on a list of items. It's far easier, and less shameful, to rate one's disclosure in regard to a short-phrased category (e.g., "my sexual fantasies") than it is to offer specific details of same, especially if this is done on a paper-and-pencil measure rather than in a face-to-face situation. Nonetheless, the results of this type of research must be understood in the context of the fact that at least some of the people some of the time will not, even on anonymous surveys, reveal intimate truths about themselves.

What did we find when we analyzed these data? As Table 3.1 indicates, among the 80 specific items on this measure, the five items with the highest scores (most thoroughly discussed) were:

> "Aspects of my personality that I dislike, worry about, or regard as a handicap."
> "Characteristics of my parents that I dislike."
> "Feelings of desperation, depression, or despair."
> "My feelings of rage or anger toward my parents."
> "My feelings of rage or anger toward my spouse/partner."

TABLE 3.1. Items Most Discussed in Therapy

	M	SD
1. The aspects of my personality that I dislike, worry about, or regard as a handicap to me	4.30	0.92
2. Characteristics of my parents that I dislike	4.24	0.98
3. Feelings of desperation, depression, or despair	4.20	0.94
4. My feelings about having my own needs met versus meeting the needs of others	4.07	1.04
5. My feelings of rage or anger toward my parents	4.06	1.00
6. My feelings of rage or anger toward my partner/spouse	4.05	1.0
7. My feelings about my achievements to this point in my life	4.03	0.98
8. My reaction to others' criticism of me	4.01	1.00
9. My expectations and hopes for the future	4.01	1.00
10. My feelings at being rejected by a spouse or lover	3.99	1.15
11. My feelings about my friends	3.98	1.04

Note. Items were scored on a 5-point scale where 1 = not discussed, and 5 = discussed thoroughly. From Hall and Farber (2001). Copyright 2001 by *The Journal of the American Academy of Psychoanalysis.* Reprinted by permission of The Guilford Press.

TABLE 3.2. Items Least Discussed in Therapy

	M	SD
1. My sexual feelings toward or sexual fantasies about my therapist	1.76	1.11
2. My interest in pornographic books, magazines, movies, videos, etc.	1.82	1.14
3. Bathroom habits: extreme fastidiousness, compulsive regularity or habitual irregularity, etc.	1.90	1.25
4. My experience of or feelings about masturbation	2.09	1.30
5. Aspects of my body that I am most satisfied with	2.15	1.17
6. My nervous habits, such as nail biting or hair twirling	2.17	1.28
7. My experience of or feelings about menstruation, including premenstrual syndrome	2.19	1.30
8. The time I lost my virginity; what it meant to me	2.19	1.47
9. My sexual fantasies	2.20	1.25
10. My tendency to lie or distort my experience to other people	2.32	1.21

Note. Items were scored on a 5-point scale where 1 = not discussed, and 5 = discussed thoroughly. From Hall and Farber (2001). Copyright 2001 by *The Journal of the American Academy of Psychoanalysis.* Reprinted by permission of The Guilford Press.

Thus, we found that patients discuss most extensively their disappointment and frustration with themselves and those closest to them. Stated somewhat differently, patients are most prone to discussing feelings of frustration, depression, and anger toward perceived inadequacies in themselves, their parents, and their spouse or partner. Orlinsky and Howard (1975), as part of their seminal investigation into typical therapeutic experiences, found that patients most often talk about feelings and attitudes about themselves, social activities and relationships with friends and acquaintances, and relationships with significant others. Contemporary findings, then, are quite consonant with the research of nearly 30 years ago—a testament, perhaps, to the enduring nature of basic psychological concerns, at least within American society.

These findings are also consistent with Frank's (1974) idea that patients come to psychotherapy in a state of demoralization—their way of making sense of their world no longer works, leaving them disillusioned and despairing. They come to therapy to examine their flaws and damaged sense of self. Furthermore, they come to discuss their feelings toward their parents and significant others. Consistent with stereotypical notions of therapy, patients tend to speak angrily about their parents, assumedly blaming them for some of their own problems. Spouses and partners also seem to be frequent targets of patient venom, providing some credence to spouses' fears and fantasies that therapy is often a forum for marital complaints and blame. This may reflect the well-documented phenomenon that the experience of shame is often accompanied by attempts to externalize blame (e.g., Tangney, 1990; Tangney, Wagner, Fletcher, & Gramazow, 1992).

Discussion in therapy of angry feelings toward parents or spouse, or one's reaction to others' criticisms (another highly endorsed item), likely reflects not just individuals' sense of impaired agency but also their sense of impaired communion with others—parents and significant others who have failed them in some way, prior significant others who have rejected them, friends and family who have been overly critical. Apparently, both of these primary existential concerns—who I am (identity) and who I am with others (intimacy)—are central issues in therapy. In fact, another highly endorsed item—my feelings about having my needs met versus meeting the needs of others—explicitly reflects the tension between these two issues.

WHAT ISSUES DO PATIENTS AVOID DISCUSSING IN PSYCHOTHERAPY?

As Table 3.2 indicates, items with the lowest mean scores in this research included "my sexual feelings toward or sexual fantasies about my therapist," "my interest in pornographic books, magazines, movies, videos, etc.," and "bathroom habits." Whereas some sexual issues, including "the nature of my sexual experiences" (mean of 3.2 on a 7-point scale) and even "my sexual affairs, either while I was married or while I was involved with someone who expected me to be faithful" (mean of 3.2), are discussed with a fair amount of detail, many others tend to be avoided. Discussion in therapy of pornographic interests or of sexual feelings toward one's therapist tends especially to be unaddressed, seemingly reflecting some deeply held ideas in this culture regarding the boundaries of appropriate disclosures. Pattee and Farber (2004) recently confirmed these earlier findings, reporting that discussion of sexual feelings toward one's therapist was the lowest rated item in their study. While we might speculate that, over time, patients would become more at ease with discussing many sexual issues, there is also the possibility that the opposite might occur. McWilliams (1994), it will be remembered, contends that discussion of sexual issues in therapy actually becomes more difficult as patients develop strong emotional reactions to their therapists.

How is it possible, some might ask, that long-term psychotherapy patients avoid talking extensively about sex? One possibility is that those asking this question have not accurately remembered the frequency or intensity of discussions of sex in either their own therapy or those of their patients, instead focusing on (and thus overrepresenting) a few memorable occasions. But the stronger likelihood is that this finding represents a good example of the typical therapeutic paradox: that, while many patients do discuss sex to a moderate degree, they also leave out a fair amount. These issues, after all, are those that especially evoke shame and resistance. This finding also brings to mind the common tendency for patients to resist extensive discussion of difficult material by focusing on related issues that are more easily addressed and at least moderately salient. As Kahn et al. (2001) have noted, "Frequent disclosures of non-distressing content may actually serve as barriers to client progress, particularly if they detract from the client's presenting issue" (p. 204).

One surprise regarding least discussed issues was that money ("the importance and meaning of money to me"), an issue often considered taboo, was found not to be especially difficult for patients to discuss in therapy. This may represent something unique about American culture, or it may simply reflect the fact that this item was worded in very general terms. Arguably, had the item been phrased to include specifics about how much money an individual actually makes, or his or her net worth, findings might have been different.

Many of the items omitted from analysis in these studies (due to insufficient numbers of individuals supplying data) reflect the related themes of violence and abuse, for example, "my experience of beating and raping someone," "my experience of sexually abusing my children or children entrusted to my care." These themes have been found by others (Norton et al., 1974; Weiner & Shuman, 1984) to be prominent among issues typically withheld in therapy.

At this point, what may be obvious is that client failure to discuss certain issues in depth may stem from quite disparate circumstances. For the most part, I've attributed this phenomenon to conscious inhibition, typically a function of shame or fear of addressing certain thoughts and feelings. But the most parsimonious explanation for why clients don't discuss certain issues in great depth is simply because these issues are not of great import to them. As one patient remarked to me following my inquiry into a new area of his life: "I'm here to discuss just one issue—I don't want to talk about my whole life." If a patient, then, fails to talk about his brother in therapy, it may mean that he's avoiding an important issue that's been on his mind; or it may simply mean that he gets along reasonably well with his brother, has no particular need to address this in therapy, and wants to address more problematic concerns.

In addition, some patients choose not to disclose extensively (or at all) about certain issues because this decision may be quite effective in alleviating anxiety. Employing very different research strategies, multiple investigators have shown that when palliatives, such as denial and avoiding negative thoughts, don't prevent adaptive action, they may reduce distress (Bonanno et al., 1995; Folkman & Lazarus, 1988; Kelly, 1998, 2000; Taylor & Brown, 1988).

Overall, how much do patients disclose? The overall mean disclosure score in this first group of studies (Farber & Hall, 2002; Hall & Farber, 2001) was 3.2, corresponding closely to the midpoint on the 5-point scale. That is, summed over a broad range of moderately to highly intimate topics, these patients indicated that they disclosed to a moderate extent. Other indications that most patients find therapy a generally safe place to discuss the key issues in their lives come from several other studies by my research team (Berano & Farber, 2006; Farber & Sohn, 1997; Pattee & Farber, 2004; Sohn & Farber, 2003). In response to the question "Overall, how self-disclosing have you been to your therapist?," patients' mean scores in these studies have ranged from 5.5 to 5.9 (on a 7-point scale). Similarly, in response to the question "What percentage of 'who you truly are' have you revealed to your therapist?," patients' average scores have been between 79 and 82 on a 1–100 scale.[1] Thus, while research clearly indicates that they keep secrets from their therapists, patients nonetheless see themselves as highly self-disclosing. That is, these results again suggest that patients are simultaneously both self-disclosing and secretive. The implicit message from patients seems to be "I will tell you a great deal about myself, but I will not tell you everything."

FACTORS THAT AFFECT PATIENT DISCLOSURE IN PSYCHOTHERAPY

Drawing on case material and theoretical reports, the preceding chapter reviewed a number of factors thought to influence patient disclosure. Research has now begun to weigh in on this issue. For example, studies conducted by my research team (e.g., Farber & Hall, 2002; Hall & Farber, 2001; Pattee & Farber, 2004) have investigated the effects on disclosure of several variables, especially gender.

Research has consistently found gender differences in disclosure in nontherapeutic situations. For example, Jourard's early work (1971a, 1971b) indicated that women typically disclose more personal information than men. Furthermore, a meta-analysis of 205 studies of sex differences in

---

[1] But this is a difficult statistic to interpret: As one respondent wrote on the questionnaire, "I've revealed 100% of the 40% that I know myself." That is, it is hard to determine, from the way the question was asked, whether these clients were "keeping" 20% of themselves to themselves—assumedly their most intimate 20%—or whether they were revealing 100% of the 80% of themselves that they knew and could reveal. Moreover, because these clients were still in therapy, this percentage could increase over time. Regardless of the exact interpretation, however, this set of statistics does suggest that these clients believe that they are highly disclosing and that their therapists know them well, if not completely.

self-disclosure (Dindia & Allen, 1992) confirmed this conclusion, finding that women tend to disclose more than men in both same-sex and cross-sex dyads, albeit only slightly. In contrast, in a study focused specifically on the therapeutic situation, Weiner and Shuman (1984) found that women disclose less than men and that women most often withhold discussion of sexual material whereas men are more reluctant to discuss issues related to violence. Unfortunately, much of the recent empirical work in the area of client disclosure (Hill et al., 1992, 1993; Kelly, 1998) has utilized relatively small sample sizes, and no gender differences were analyzed in these studies.

In our studies, we found no difference in overall mean disclosure between men and women, nor any overall difference in the extent of difficulty they find in discussing intimate topics in therapy. Furthermore, we found that men and women share many of the same concerns. As Table 3.3 indicates, both men and women appear to be interested in discussing aspects of their personality that they dislike, characteristics of their parents that they dislike, and their achievements to this point in their lives. For women, the most thoroughly discussed issue was "feelings of desperation,

TABLE 3.3. A Gender Comparison of Items Most Discussed in Therapy

Female respondents	Male respondents
1. Feelings of desperation, depression, or despair ($M = 4.29$, $SD = .84$)	1. The aspects of my personality that I dislike, worry about, or regard as a handicap to me ($M = 4.39$, $SD = .84$)
2. Aspects of my personality that I dislike, worry about, or regard as a handicap to me ($M = 4.26$, $SD = .95$)	2. Characteristics of my parents that I dislike ($M = 4.22$, $SD = 1.07$)
3. Characteristics of my parents that I dislike ($M = 4.25$, $SD = .94$)	3. My feelings about my achievements to this point in my life ($M = 4.17$, $SD = .91$)
4. My feelings of rage or anger toward my parents ($M = 4.13$, $SD = .95$)	4. My feelings about having my own needs met versus meeting the needs of other people ($M = 4.09$, $SD = 1.04$)
5. My feelings of rage or anger toward my spouse/partner ($M = 4.09$, $SD = .98$)	5. My sense of pride in who I am and what I can do ($M = 4.0$, $SD = .99$)

Note. Items were scored on a 5-point scale in which 1 = not discussed and 5 = discussed thoroughly. From Farber (2003). Copyright 2003 by John Wiley & Sons, Inc. This material is used by permission of John Wiley & Sons, Inc.

depression, or despair"; for men, it was aspects of their personality that they dislike.

Furthermore, as Table 3.4 indicates, among the least discussed items for both groups are interest in pornography (the lowest-ranked item for women) and sexual fantasies about one's therapist (the second-lowest ranked item for men). There were only 3 items (of 80 total) on which women had significantly higher disclosure scores: "My desire for children—my feelings that I may not be able to have them, either for physical reasons or because I will not find a mate"; "The nature of my sexual experiences"; and, not surprisingly, "My experience of or feelings about menstruation, including premenstrual syndrome." The single item on which men's disclosure scores significantly exceeded women's was "My interest in pornographic books, magazines, movies, videos, etc."

Thus, while popular culture often expounds the notion that women are more relational and self-disclosing than men, in our studies overall disclosure for men and women was equivalent, and there was even a great degree of overlap regarding the most and least thoroughly discussed issues. The most conspicuous exceptions—that women are more likely to extensively discuss issues regarding menstruation and their desire for children—are quite consonant not only with gender role expectations but biological imperatives. One of our studies (Pattee & Farber, 2004) did find

TABLE 3.4. A Gender Comparison of Items Least Discussed in Therapy

Female respondents	Male respondents
1. My interest in pornographic books, magazines, movies, videos, etc. ($M = 1.58$, $SD = .97$)	1. My experience of, or feelings about menstruation, including PMS ($M = 1.54$, $SD = .82$)
2. My sexual feelings toward or sexual fantasies about my therapist ($M = 1.67$, $SD = 1.09$)	2. My sexual feelings toward or sexual fantasies about my therapist ($M = 1.97$, $SD = 1.13$)
3. Bathroom habits, extreme fastidiousness, compulsive regularity or habitual irregularity, etc. ($M = 1.85$, $SD = 1.20$)	3. Bathroom habits, extreme fastidiousness, compulsive regularity, or habitual irregularity, etc. ($M = 1.97$, $SD = 1.35$
4. My experience of or feelings about masturbation ($M = 1.99$, $SD = 1.32$)	4. Nervous habits, such as nail biting or hair twirling ($M = 1.98$, $SD = 1.23$)
5. My sexual fantasies ($M = 2.06$, $SD = 1.26$)	5. Aspects of my body that I am most satisfied with ($M = 2.04$, $SD = 1.12$)

Note. Items were scored on a 5-point scale in which 1 = not discussed and 5 = discussed thoroughly.

that women with female therapists had greater difficulty discussing intimate topics in therapy than either men with female therapists or women with male therapists.

The absence of extensive gender influences may reflect the fact that participants in our early studies had been with their current therapist an average of 37 months; widespread differences based on gender may have been attenuated by the familiarity and comfort established over a lengthy period of therapy. It is also possible that men who enter treatment are already in violation of the social injunction against males asking for help; thus, they may constitute a distinct subgroup with different expectations and values regarding autonomy and disclosure. That is, although it may be more difficult for men to enter therapy, once there they may have no more difficulty availing themselves of the opportunities provided by therapy than women. Relatedly, a significant proportion of the men in these studies were themselves mental health professionals, and thus likely to have been socialized, through graduate training, to accept and even endorse the process of disclosure as a means toward health and growth. But the lack of gender differences in disclosure may also reflect the fact that, as Harry Stack Sullivan once observed, "We are all more human than otherwise." In short, despite the intense focus in recent decades on cognitive and emotional differences in the way that men and women process and react to life events—a focus that extends from serious research to newsstand magazines to endless riffs on popular sitcoms—within the confines of the therapist's office, men and women tend to discourse on the same universally troubling concerns.

We also investigated several other factors that we thought might influence the disclosure process. For example, we found that length of time in therapy and strength of the therapeutic alliance predicted overall disclosure in therapy. Clearly, the longer a person is in therapy with the same therapist, the more opportunity he or she has to disclose. That is, over time, most patients, except for those most "stuck" or resistant, both broaden the domain of issues broached with their therapist and intensify the depth of discussion of those focal topics that are most relevant to their lives. Moreover, this finding, like that of the *Consumer Reports* study (Seligman, 1995), speaks to the added value of longer-term therapy. Many patients apparently benefit from the opportunities offered in longer open-ended therapies to further discuss and process old material as well as to uncover and understand new material. Many patients, then, do not reach asymptote in terms of their depth of disclosure; rather, they continue over time to further their self-exploration through the use of therapy.

That the therapeutic alliance is a significant predictor of disclosure lends support to the argument that it is the single most potent variable in the therapeutic process (Horvath & Bedi, 2002). The results of our research suggest that an effective therapeutic alliance not only is mutative in itself (by allowing clients to interact with an empathic and caring other) but also facilitates an atmosphere in which increased disclosure occurs, which, in turn, offers opportunities for new means of understanding and coping with deeply felt issues. In fact, patients who report better working alliances with their therapists tend to report less of a discrepancy between the extent of their discussion of key psychotherapeutic issues and the importance they assign to these issues. Furthermore, patients who report feeling more connected to their therapists during moments of self-disclosure also perceive their treatment to have been more successful (Pattee & Farber, 2004).

We also investigated patient shame and found its relationship to disclosure to be somewhat less robust than anticipated. That is, we failed to find a significant relationship between client shame proneness and overall disclosure. Nevertheless, shame did emerge as a significant predictor of disclosure on a cluster of items associated with negative affect. Clients with a greater tendency to shame were less likely to discuss feelings of self-loathing, perceptions of personal failure, personality aspects that they dislike, and events in their past about which they are most ashamed. This finding is quite consistent with a study that found that patients' nondisclosure of distressful feelings (e.g., guilt, hatred, disgust) was related to the thought that telling would engender shame (Macdonald & Morley, 2001). Thus, not surprisingly, it appears that shame becomes more prominent a factor in the decision to disclose as the nature of what is being disclosed becomes more personally distressing.

THE QUESTION OF SALIENCE

Left unanswered by much of the research reported in this chapter thus far is the issue of importance: Where on the continuum of relevance–triviality do patients' disclosures and nondisclosures lie? Clearly, some patient discourse is close to the heart of the matter, central to a person's sense of self and deeply connected to the reasons that this person has sought out therapy. As noted earlier, however, other discourse seems to be mostly in the service of resistance—speech with the primary purpose of avoiding discussion of far more serious, if difficult-to-address, issues. As one patient of mine once remarked: "I could talk here forever, as long as I don't have to talk about anything important." There is, then, a critical distinction between failing to discuss a topic of great personal import and failing to discuss a topic of limited relevance. In this vein, my research team (Farber & Sohn, 1997) posed the following question: For which issues do the greatest discrepancies exist between personal importance or salience and extent of discussion in therapy?

To investigate this matter, we asked 50 patients (mean age 35; in therapy, on average, for slightly over 5 years) to indicate not only the extent to which they had discussed each of 101 moderately to highly intimate topics with their therapist but also the extent to which they considered each topic relevant or salient to them. The two-part procedure—of having clients rate disclosure as well as relevance—makes possible the identification of those topics for which the greatest and smallest discrepancies exist between disclosure and personal relevance. "Discrepancy scores" represent the difference on each item between ratings of disclosure and ratings of personal salience.

Items with the highest positive discrepancy scores (i.e., those with higher disclosure scores than salience scores) included "feelings of wanting to seriously harm someone," "fantasies of revenge against those who have hurt me," and "feelings of self-loathing." These are the items about which clients are essentially indicating "I talk more about this subject than its importance warrants." One possibility here is that these items are somewhat impulse-driven and tied more to the immediacy of feelings experienced during a given therapy session than to long-term conflicts.

Items for which there were large negative discrepancies between self-disclosure and salience were "my feelings of inadequacy or failure," "concerns about my sexual performance," "my experience or feelings about masturbation," "my experiences of being sexually abused as a child," and "the nature of my sexual experiences." These are the items about which clients are implicitly acknowledging "I should be speaking more about this in therapy." While it is important to remember that these items are discussed to a certain extent, it is nonetheless surprising that there is still apparently a reluctance to fully explore sexual issues with one's therapist. Perhaps to a greater extent than with other issues, discussion of sexual issues and abuse-related issues proceeds slowly and with much reticence.

CONCLUSIONS

In summary, research indicates that, whereas most patients disclose deeply personal experiences in therapy, a significant proportion consciously conceal some significant information. Even in planned terminations following a lengthy depth-oriented treatment, some material will inevitably remain unprocessed. Arguably, this may even be somewhat helpful. As Regan and Hill (1992) suggested, some secrecy may facilitate patients' internalization of benignly influential therapeutic interventions. That is, it may help patients become their own therapists and carry on therapeutic work alone, in between sessions and after therapy is terminated (Geller, Cooley, & Hartley, 1982; Geller & Farber, 1993). In addition, as noted earlier, keeping some material private may be a way for patients to maintain a strong sense of self. It may reflect the more general need to balance the tension between the need for autonomy and the need for relatedness.

Research findings also show that there are several categories of nondisclosed information (secrets, thoughts and feelings left unsaid, and client reactions to their therapists); that patients tend to withhold immediately experienced negative reactions from their therapists; that disliked characteristics of oneself and parents are among the most thoroughly discussed issues, whereas certain aspects of sex, aggression, and personal failure tend to be avoided; that men and women disclose to the same general extent and on similar topics; that shame inhibits disclosure of negative affect; and that a strong therapeutic alliance, overall tendency to be disclosing, and time in therapy all facilitate disclosure.

Research and clinical reports indicate that the task of disclosing to another is invariably more difficult than patients anticipate and inevitably proceeds at a nonlinear pace with periods of both surprising resistance and remarkable productivity. As has been emphasized repeatedly throughout these pages, for most patients there is an ongoing struggle between the desire to be known fully, both to oneself and another, and the simultaneous desire to protect oneself from the shame and vulnerability of having one's most base instincts, experiences, and fantasies fully exposed. Although self-report measures that focus solely upon patient verbal discourse miss much of what is actually communicated (i.e., nonverbally), therapists do need to be sensitive to issues that are difficult for most patients to speak about even in the safety of the therapeutic setting.

I imagine that most clinicians (especially those who are psychodynamically oriented) would posit a significant relationship between the extent of client disclosure and outcome, and some empirical studies have supported this conclusion. Nevertheless, there is growing debate in the therapeutic community over whether disclosure does, in fact, inexorably lead to improvement, and it is this topic that is the focus of the next chapter.

CHAPTER 4

Patient Disclosure

The Outcome Controversy

> To express unafraid and unashamed what one really thinks and feels is one of the great consolations of life.
> —REIK (cited in Seldes, 1985, p. 385)

> I do conceal as much as possible of those thoughts that are not meant to be shared. You wonder about a conversation with nothing concealed—its real name is hell, I believe.
> —YALOM (1992, p. 92)

In Chapter 1, I introduced the debate over whether expression or repression is the best option in the aftermath of traumatic events. In this chapter, concerns about the value of disclosure will be revisited in the specific context of psychotherapy.

The question of whether disclosure in psychotherapy is beneficial or harmful has raged since the early days of Freud but has been reintroduced recently into the public's consciousness by vigorous debates over the value of psychotherapy for victims of terrorist attacks and natural disasters. Supporters of psychotherapy believe strongly in the value of talking about such experiences as a means of healing current wounds and of reducing the potential for future stress-related problems; critics claim that encouraging victims of trauma to talk about their experiences has the strong potential for retraumatizing them. As noted earlier, there is considerable evidence (clinical, philosophical, and empirical) to support both positions, and, indeed, the ultimate verdict will likely be "it depends."

To review for a moment: The need for and value of disclosure are almost certainly a function of multiple variables, including patients' goals and values; the nature, relevance, and timing of what is disclosed; and the therapeutic relationship in which the disclosure unfolds. Perhaps most basically, the value of disclosure depends on the characteristic ways that each person best copes with stress. Some people ("sensitizers") find relief in revealing personal information; others ("repressors") do not. Paraphrasing the Eagles' perspicacious observation in their song "Hotel California," some of us dance to remember and some to forget. In fact, Kahn et al. (2001) essentially confirmed this observation, finding that those high on the trait of "distress disclosure" were more likely to evidence decreases in perceived stress and symptomatology over the course of counseling. That is, some individuals are likely to benefit more from their disclosures than others.

Still, there is a strong belief among most clinicians, especially those who practice within a psychodynamic framework, that talking about problems helps. Although it wasn't Freud but rather his patient, Anna O, who dubbed the process "the talking cure," this appellation stuck because it captured so well the essential assumption of therapeutic work—that talking about problems eases one's mind and alleviates manifest symptomatology. Even therapeutic approaches that don't emphasize a disclosure–awareness–change link implicitly consider patient disclosure the core activity of psychotherapy, the center from which all therapist interventions emanate (Stiles, 1995).

Furthermore, it seems safe to assume that most individuals who seek out psychotherapeutic services believe that the process of disclosing to another will be helpful. Many expect to reveal deeply personal material to their therapists out of a conviction (shared, of course, by the therapist) that doing so will make them feel better. And many, though not all, will be glad to have done so. In fact, many patients rehearse what they will say to their therapists, eager to share new thoughts, memories, and feelings.

But, as I've stated in earlier chapters, there is another side of this debate, one that emphasizes the potential for disclosure to exacerbate distress. Thus, alongside appreciative words from patients, all therapists have also heard this lament or a variation thereof: "It's enough already—the more I talk about this the worse I feel." Or: "OK, we've been there, I understand it, I've talked about it forever and I still don't feel better." Or this refrain, one heard repeatedly in the wake of traumatic events, including those of 9/11: "You don't understand. You keep wanting me to discuss this as if that'll help. I want to forget this, not remember it any better."

Some individuals do seem to believe that "some things are better not seen nor talked about" or "I don't want to ever go there again." Dostoyevsky expressed this notion in *The Idiot* (1868): "By digging into our souls, we often dig up what might better have remained there unnoticed" (p. 140). In his novel *When Nietzche Wept* (1992), Yalom noted that "despair is the price one pays for self-awareness" (p. 139). And one of the characters in Kazantzakis' beautifully crafted book *Zorba the Greek* (1952) says: "Let people be, boss; don't open their eyes. And supposing you did, what'd they see? Their misery! Leave their eyes closed, boss, and let them go on dreaming!" (p. 61).

Writing from a clinical rather than literary perspective, Levinson, Sharaf, and Gilbert (1966) found that focusing on one's inner life and painful memories serves to keep experiences of shame and anxiety in the forefront of consciousness. Providing some empirical support for these ideas, a study of the effects of psychological-mindedness in individuals—that is, the tendency to reflect on the meaning and motivation of behavior, thoughts, and feelings in oneself and others—concluded that individuals with high scores on this trait were essentially "wiser but sadder" (Farber, 1989). Such individuals strive to deepen their understanding of themselves and others and embrace this trait, believing that it enriches them and their relationships with others. But they also acknowledge that their awareness of inner pain and suffering, of the tragic elements in life, suffuses their sense of the world. They tend to believe that this is a price worth paying for the richness of their intrapsychic and interpersonal lives, but clearly not everyone subscribes to this view. There are many individuals (e.g., repressors) who do not believe in the psychological benefits of discussing and understanding sorrow and pain.

Thus, despite many psychotherapists' bias toward baring one's soul in the pursuit of self-awareness and emotional health, there is ample support for being cautious or otherwise inclined. Indeed, it could be argued that the popularity of antidepressant medications and even of cognitive-behavioral therapies speaks to the needs of those who prefer their pain to be ameliorated in ways other than unfolding that which has been repressed, forgotten, or secreted away. For these individuals, the process of self-disclosure may seem unconnected or even antithetical to the process of change. Thus, there are individuals who seem to need to continually discuss and address their experiences in order to make continuing sense of what seems to be inexplicable and those who feel instead that they need—indeed must—forget in order to go on. To the extent that individuals vary in this regard, it makes the task of determining the general value of disclosure in therapy all the more difficult. That is, in aggregating the results of studies examining the effects of disclosure, it is easy to forget that a small positive effect may be the result of combining data from two disparate groups: those who experience strong positive benefits from disclosure and those who experience either no effects or negative effects from their disclosures.

PENNEBAKER'S STUDIES

Let us return to the work of James Pennebaker, whose studies on the healing effects of disclosure have been both influential and controversial.

Unlike most of the work of academic psychologists, his has reached popular audiences. In part, this is because his major finding—that writing about trauma is effective in reducing distress—is one that has resonated with large groups of individuals across all segments of our culture. It is a prescription that is at once simple, effective, and nonmedical. It can be done whenever one wants, without appointment, and has, moreover, the virtue of a self-applied intervention. It is firmly within the bounds of self-help and yet comes with the imprimatur of scientific approval. Its controversy essentially resides in its being touted (though not by Pennebaker himself) as a means to heal traumatic wounds effectively, permanently, and in all individuals. In this sense, it may take its place alongside a long list of psychological interventions whose early promise led to exaggerated claims by enthusiastic proponents that, under the sway of empirical evidence, ultimately gave way to far more modest and temperate conclusions (e.g., eye movement desensitization and reprocessing [EMDR]).

According to Pennebaker (1997), "The mere act of disclosure is a powerful therapeutic agent that may account for a substantial percentage of variance in the healing process" (p. 162). While his studies have not involved psychotherapy patients, the work is often cited as offering indirect evidence for the efficacy of disclosure in clinical situations. Thus, a summary of this work should serve as helpful background material for understanding current controversies about the value of disclosure in psychotherapy.

The basic paradigm is remarkably simple: Write (at a minimum) 3–5 days, in any way, on any emotionally stressful experience for a minimum time (e.g., 20 minutes). Keep the writing samples private; do not share what you've written. You will not get feedback. Abide by a "flip-out" rule—if it starts feeling bad, stop writing. Another way of stating this: Allow self-dosing and go only as far as you are able.

As of 2002, more than 100 studies employing this paradigm had been carried out, and, according to Pennebaker (2002), 60–70% had replicated the very positive results of his first group of studies. There are improvements in terms of physical health and immune system functioning; there are a reduced number of visits to a physician and fewer days taken off from work. Workers laid off from jobs who disclosed through writing have found jobs more quickly than those who did not write. Recently Sloan and Marx (2004) documented a reduction in depressive symptomatology among individuals with moderate PTSD symptoms. Among others, those shown to have benefited from this paradigm include students, prisoners, Holocaust survivors, and individuals with breast and prostate cancer. The paradigm has been shown to be effective in countries with quite disparate cultures, including Mexico, Japan, Spain, Italy, the Netherlands, and New Zealand. In his review of this research, Smyth (1998) concluded that there was a "medium" effect size for health benefits that accrue as a result of writing about trauma, a 23% greater improvement in the writing groups as compared to control groups. Sheese, Brown, and Graziano (2004) found that these beneficial health outcomes could even be realized through writing about traumatic experiences in emails.

Pennebaker suggests that the strategy of writing about trauma is particularly effective for people who say that they're thinking about the trauma too much and for people who continue to talk about the event several weeks afterward but have not benefited from talking. Telling the same story to either themselves or others means they are stuck; they often benefit by changing at least some elements in the story as they write about it. Writing about trauma may also be especially useful for those who don't have a social network in which to discuss the event in an accepting, receptive way. And finally, this strategy may be helpful in cases where the story is too embarrassing or shameful to share with others.

Why does it work? According to Pennebaker (2002), there are several possibilities, many of which overlap with the benefits of talking about trauma with another. There's the phenomenon of taking control of an otherwise out-of-control situation. That is, the individual controls how much he or she talks or writes about a frightening situation and, in doing so, may gradually—at his or her own pace—become desensitized to the toxic feelings and thoughts. The initially overwhelming feelings lose their power to overwhelm. Similarly, Bootzin (1997) suggests that repeated writing results in the extinction of the connection between memories and distress. There is also the benefit of cognitively processing a complex event, of making sense of or finding meaning in something previously inchoate. Stiles (1995) speaks of this as "assimilating" previously split-off problematic experiences. I noted this phenomenon earlier in a discussion of how disclosure to a therapist could help an individual find a new perspective on an unresolved issue, a coherent narrative that allows him or her to make more peace with what happened. In this regard, too, I like what the poet W. H. Auden had to say: "I look at what I write so that I can see what I think" (cited in Rosen & Krotov, 2005, p. 3).

There is also the possibility that the Pennebaker task is effective because it increases one's working memory—as a consequence of writing about trauma, one no longer has to be so preoccupied with these events or, conversely, expend considerable energy trying not to think of them (thought suppression). Inhibition, as several researchers have noted, requires work. In this vein, Borkovek, Roemer, and Kenyon (1995) have hypothesized that disclosure and worrying constitute opposite sides of the "emotional processing coin." Writing about or discussing traumatic material may free up cognitive and emotional "space." In addition, some have suggested a social integration hypothesis: that, in writing for another (regardless of the fact that the other won't read the work), one forges some social connection, or at least eschews total social isolation. There is also the complementary hypothesis: that writ-

ing enables individuals to disclose without fear of negative social consequences—that is, it may provide an avenue for disclosure when interpersonal
expression is not viable or seems too frightening (Smyth, 1998). Finally,
Pennebaker (1995) suggests that following an emotionally charged disclosure an individual's biological, social, cognitive and emotional functioning is
more harmonious, that "all features of mind and body become synchronous"
(p. 8).

PATIENT DISCLOSURE
AND PSYCHOTHERAPY OUTCOME:
WHAT DOES THE RESEARCH SAY?

There is overwhelming evidence that writing about trauma is helpful. However, there is at best an inexact parallel between this task and that of psychotherapy. Arguably the primary difference is that one is a private task
that involves writing, whereas the other is an interpersonal task that primarily involves speaking. Another basic difference is in the players: One
involves research subjects (most often college students), the other real psychotherapy patients. In fact, psychotherapy patients are often those who
have failed to benefit from disclosing to a nonprofessional other (Frank,
1974). Yet another difference lies in the focus of the tasks: One paradigm
directs its attention to trauma, the other to a wide variety of perceived difficulties, including trauma but not limited to this experience.

Thus, in contrast to the consistent evidence of the benefits of written
disclosure, research has tended to be equivocal regarding the relationship
of patient disclosure to psychotherapy outcome. Studies of disclosure in
group therapy (e.g., Anchor & Sandler, 1973; Bennun & Schindler, 1988;
Freedman & Enright, 1996) have shown that patient disclosure is positively correlated with treatment outcome. In addition, the majority of
findings of individual treatment studies demonstrate either a positive or a
nonsignificant correlation between the two variables (e.g., Kahn et al.,
2001).

Still, a fair amount of research has demonstrated mixed results. Illus-
trative of this trend, Regan and Hill (1992) found that, while the overall
number and valence of "things left unsaid" by clients was not related to
outcome, the content of what was left unsaid was significantly related to
outcome. Specifically, the more feeling-related observations left unsaid by
clients—for example, "I wasn't able to express all my feelings articulately"
(p. 169)—the less clients experienced sessions as deep and the less satisfied
they were with treatment. Similarly, several studies by my own research
team have yielded mixed results. One study (Farber & Sohn, 2001) found
that overall disclosure in therapy was not related to outcome but that
salience of disclosure (i.e., an indication that clients were talking about

what was important to them) was related to positive outcome. On the other hand, a second study (Sohn & Farber, 2003) found the opposite: that salience of disclosure was not related to outcome but that overall disclosure was positively related to outcome. And a third study (Pattee & Farber, 2004) was unable to find a significant relationship between outcome and either salience or extent of disclosure.

Stiles and colleagues have generally found either no signification relationship between disclosure and outcome or a negative relationship. For example, Stiles (1984) found no significant associations between the extent of client disclosure and client-, therapist-, and outsider-rated "depth" of the session, but also reported that sessions that were rated as high in client disclosure by outside raters were seen as especially rough and unpleasant. Stiles' research group also reported that client self-disclosure was not significantly correlated with any of a variety of outcome measures (McDaniel, Stiles, & McGaughey, 1981) and that the extent of disclosure was not predictive of improvement within either a directive or more exploratory type of therapy (Stiles & Shapiro, 1994).

The high degree of inconsistency in the literature is likely related to the diverse ways in which self-disclosure and outcome have been operationalized. Kahn et al. (2001) contend that the relationship between disclosure and outcome in psychotherapy has been obscured by researchers' failure to differentiate between distressing and nondistressing content and between disclosure as a state (an episodic event) and a trait (a general disposition). In addition, inconsistent outcome results may be understood in terms of the aforementioned variability in patient needs and preferences: Some like disclosing and tend to benefit from this activity, some do not. Furthermore, the determination of outcome in key studies has varied in terms of whose perception was assessed (client, therapist, or outside rater), the time at which it was assessed (immediately postdisclosure or at a later point of time), and the nature of the putative benefit (e.g., symptom reduction, or perceived value or depth of therapy session). In regard to this last point, while Farber and Sohn (2001) failed to find a significant relationship between disclosure and an overall outcome measure, they did find a positive relationship between disclosure and increased patient self-understanding.

But arguably of even greater importance than these issues is the failure of virtually all studies in this area to discriminate between disclosure that is essentially ruminative (going over old material the same old ways) and disclosure that leads to new ways of understanding or framing issues. The former is likely to lead to no improvement or even negative therapeutic results, whereas the latter paradigm has a high probability for positive results. Research in the field of trauma strongly supports this argument. In their review of this research, Taylor, Kemeny, Reed, Bower, and Gruenewald (2000) underscored the "potentially deleterious effects that ruminative thought can have in the absence of finding meaning in the event" (p. 105).

Their findings suggest an important and often overlooked aspect of the psychotherapeutic process: that the goal of patient disclosure must go beyond "getting it out" to making new sense of what's always been in there. While it might be argued that good therapists have always intuitively understood this, virtually all clinicians doing long-term work have had the experience of working with patients who seem to be stuck going over the same material in the same ways for long periods of time.

Bucci's (1997) work suggests another reason why disclosure studies in psychotherapy have failed to yield consistently positive results. According to her multiple code theory, psychopathology results from the failure of integration of emotional schemas. Thus, patient disclosure cannot lead to therapeutic benefit if it has not catalyzed strong primary affect; in fact, the intensity of the affect accompanying disclosure is far more important than the content of the disclosure per se. Effective disclosure, she contends, is that which activates subsymbolic bodily and sensory experiences in psychotherapeutic sessions. Such experiences are effective precisely because they lead to changes in the emotional meaning of prior sensory experiences. Taken together with research (see above) that has emphasized the importance of discovering fresh meanings in verbal discourse, Bucci's work leads to the hypothesis that disclosure in psychotherapy is most effective (or perhaps only effective) when it leads inexorably to cognitive and/or emotional restructuring of old, ineffective narrative structures.

Are there ways of understanding why some studies have found not just inconclusive evidence for the effects of disclosure but actual negative results? One explanation is embedded in the discussion in the preceding paragraphs—the possibility that ruminative discourse may lead patients to feel worse. But let's also consider the problem of negative results by examining the pattern of findings in certain studies. For example, one of the findings in Regan and Hill's (1992) study was that when emotional content was *excluded* from the session clients rated the session as more satisfactory, smooth, and deep. We might have assumed that patients who suppress negative feelings (e.g., their anger or frustration at their therapists) would be frustrated by their inability to disclose what they are experiencing. Still, Regan and Hill found otherwise. They attempted to explain this finding in two different ways. They hypothesized that clients sensed that the expression of strong feelings would make them feel too vulnerable and that the containment of such feelings provided a necessary and reassuring degree of safety. However, quite distinct from this possibility, they also suggested that this finding might be due to a statistical artifact—that sessions in which patients acknowledged withholding emotional material might also be those in which they actually expressed a great deal of emotional material. Indeed, as they note, "it is possible that sessions with more emotional content left unsaid were perceived as being better because clients dealt with more emotional material in these sessions" (p. 172).

Stiles' work also sheds light on negative findings in this literature. His "fever model" (1987, 1995) contains several essential premises but begins with an assumption similar to that expressed by Regan and Hill (1992): that people tend to disclose more when they are distressed and that disclosure reduces the distress. "The relation of Disclosure to psychological distress is analogous to the relation of fever to physical infection: both are an indicator of some underlying disturbance and part of a restorative process" (Stiles, 1995, p. 82). The model also proposes that as individuals experience distress their awareness of this experience and its accompanying sensations (including thoughts and feelings) becomes foremost in their minds, ultimately manifesting in a tendency to disclose what is occurring to them. Individuals, according to Stiles, do not immediately anticipate any benefits from disclosing, although they may come to experience some relief from this experience. "Distress helps promote Disclosure and Disclosure helps relieve distress and hence reduce the need to Disclose" (p. 83). Stiles (1995) further suggested that normal distress can be attenuated by disclosing to friends and family members. Still, because social support may not always be available, and because intense emotional distress may be refractory to what is normally offered in the way of social support, members outside one's typical social network (e.g., clergy, psychotherapists) may sometimes be needed. However, even they may not be enough to reduce the distress.

Thus, whereas a high level of distress may promote disclosure in therapy, it is unlikely to predict positive outcome. In fact, Stiles (1995) contends that the opposite is more likely to be true because the most distressed clients—those who tend to disclose the most—are also those who tend to have the poorest outcomes. "Disclosure may have a null or even negative correlation with outcome, even though it is an essential ingredient in psychotherapy. Analogously, a high fever is not a particularly good predictor of full or rapid recovery from physical infection, and inducing a fever is rarely an effective treatment" (p. 83).

KELLY'S WORK AND THE ENSUING CONTROVERSY

In a series of provocative articles, Kelly (1998, 2000; Kelly & Achter, 1995; Kelly, Kahn, & Coulter, 1996; Kelly & McKillop, 1996) challenged long-held assumptions regarding the overall positive effects of therapist disclosure. She contended that "there is no evidence that greater client disclosure in therapy is associated with long-term benefits" (2000) and, further, that "clients may benefit from hiding some undesirable aspects of themselves from their therapists" (1998, p. 50).

Kelly based these conclusions on several pieces of evidence. She noted that in Hill et al.'s (1992) study, when therapists were aware of their clients' negative reactions during sessions, clients perceived the therapists' next interventions as less helpful than when therapists were unaware of these reactions. She cited Regan and Hill's (1992) finding of a positive relationship between the proportion of statements with emotional content that clients left unsaid and clients' satisfaction with therapy and change. (It should be remembered, however, that Regan and Hill suggested that this finding might be spurious.) Kelly (1998) also noted that in Hill et al.'s (1993) study "there was no evidence that clients who kept secrets actually had greater symptomatology" (p. 51).

Kelly downplayed Pennebaker's research on the positive effects of writing about traumatic events, suggesting that this research may not generalize to psychotherapy. She also concluded from reviewing the extant research that greater disclosure has not been proven to be associated with therapy benefits. Moreover, she cited some of her own research to conclude that keeping relevant secrets in therapy is actually associated with a reduction in symptoms. For example, she pointed to her 1998 research in which she studied a sample of 42 outpatients who had been in therapy an average of 11 sessions. Although she found that clients' general tendency toward self-concealment was associated with greater symptomatology (consistent with the research of Pennebaker and others), she emphasized a different finding: "that after the analyses adjusted for clients' dispositional tendencies to keep secrets in general and to present themselves in a socially desirable manner, the clients who were keeping relevant secrets in therapy had significantly lower symptomatology scores than those who were not" (2000, pp. 54–55).

These results, according to Kelly (2000), support the idea that clients who conceal some unfavorable aspects of themselves may benefit more from therapy than those who do not. They benefit, Kelly hypothesized, because they are then better able to construct more desirable images of themselves in the presence of an important other (their therapist). They do not have to concern themselves with actual or anticipated negative feedback from their therapists about shameful behavior, thoughts, or feelings. Rather, they present themselves in a desirable fashion, elicit positive feedback from their therapist, and benefit from this loop. Conversely, claimed Kelly, high levels of openness place clients at risk for creating unwanted negative images of themselves—one of the potentially negative consequences of disclosure noted earlier in this book.

Kelly's work, based on what she terms a self-presentational model of therapy, is consistent with previous research of Shelley Taylor (e.g., Taylor & Armor, 1996; Taylor & Brown, 1988) emphasizing the positive consequences of denial. Both positions support the idea that positive views of oneself, even if somewhat illusory, promote psychological well-being. Kelly's work is also consistent with the research of Folkman and Lazarus (1988), who have touted the benefits of coping with stress via denial so long as doing so does not interfere with opportunities to directly change the situation.

Hill, Gelso, and Mohr (2000) disagreed strongly with Kelly's conclusions, particularly in regard to her contention that concealment is positively correlated with therapeutic improvement. Among other critiques of Kelly's conclusions, Hill et al. pointed to a fact alluded to earlier: that many phenomena have been included within the category of client concealment, making it difficult to generalize across studies. Furthermore, they asserted that concealment in therapy is a function of many factors and not just determined by clients' self-presentational needs:

> Clients have reported keeping secrets because of feeling deferent toward therapists, feeling ashamed or embarrassed, not being able personally to handle the disclosure, thinking that the therapist could not handle the disclosure, being afraid to express feelings, being concerned that revealing secrets would show the therapist how little progress had been made, not having enough time, not being willing to tell anyone, not being motivated to address the secret, or feeling loyalty to someone else. (p. 496)

Hill et al. (2000) hypothesized that therapeutic outcomes vary, depending on the reasons that clients fail to disclose. They suggested, for example, that when clients conceal out of a belief that certain problems are outside the domain of the therapist's expertise, the likelihood of a positive association between disclosure and outcome is high; by contrast, when clients conceal because of shame, a negative outcome is more likely. Furthermore, they indicated that Kelly's (1998) own data provide support for their views. The correlation in Kelly's study between relevant secret-keeping and self-reported symptomatology was, in fact, small and nonsignificant (–.11), achieving significance only when social desirability and tendency to conceal were controlled for. Their point here is that the simple association between concealment and outcome was nonsignificant and, in fact, in a negative direction.

There is at least one other significant flaw in Kelly's theory regarding the benign effects of concealing thoughts or feelings from one's therapist. It is her assumption that subsequent to any intimate disclosure a patient will suffer from intense shame, a feeling so debilitating that it will impair an individual's self-image. This assumption is likely incorrect—or, more accurately, overstated—for at least two reasons. First, most therapists are sufficiently skilled to attenuate, albeit not entirely eliminate, a patient's shame following a highly intimate disclosure. Most, especially those who have been trained in the past two decades, are well aware of the importance of the therapeutic relationship and have been taught and supervised within programs (regardless of therapeutic orientation) that have emphasized the need for sensitivity, empathy, and the repair of strained alliances. "Shameful" disclosures, then, are likely to be met with understanding and positive regard. Indeed, based on a small-scale study, Farber et al. (2004) concluded that "most patients feel that therapy is a safe place to disclose, made especially so by the goodness of the therapeutic relationship" (p. 340).

Second, findings from this same study provide preliminary evidence to indicate that, while shame does occur as a consequence of intimate disclosures, it tends to be only one of multiple emotions that are experienced. In fact, this study showed that other emotions tend to be far more intensely experienced by clients in the aftermath of disclosures. Clients were asked to rate, on a 7-point Likert-type scale (1 = very little; 4 = somewhat; 7 = to a great extent), the extent to which they experienced each of 10 emotions "immediately after" they had revealed something difficult to their therapist. The mean score for "ashamed" was 3.4; however, the mean scores for 7 other emotions equaled or exceeded this, including "relieved" (5.6), "vulnerable" (5.4), "authentic" (5.1), "safe" (5.1), and "proud" (4.5). Thus, Kelly's assumption that shame is the primary emotion during or immediately after client disclosures seems incorrect. Indeed, as Farber et al. (2004) found, "Although shame and vulnerability are powerful and salient emotions throughout the disclosure process, they are not the only emotional consequences of disclosure; clients also experience pride, safety, authenticity, and therapist approval" (p. 344). It may well be the case that shame is experienced far more acutely prior to difficult disclosures than in their aftermath.

CONCLUSIONS

As has been noted, research in this field has been hindered by the limitations of self-disclosure assessment instruments. For years, the industry standard had been the Jourard Self-Disclosure Questionnaire (Jourard, 1971a), an instrument that requested participants to indicate to whom they disclosed information on a variety of topics, including hobbies and interests, financial affairs, and body image. That questionnaire has not only been outdated for several decades but never was intended to assess the extent of disclosure of the type of highly intimate information that is often discussed in therapy. More recent methodologies, like those used by Kelly and by Hill and her colleagues, have assessed only what is withheld in therapy, and not what is discussed—in effect, focusing on only half the picture. In addition, Kelly's research, though of enormous heuristic value, assesses the absence or presence of a single relevant secret. This, it would seem, overly simplifies the complex pattern of disclosures and nondisclosure in therapy. My own work, although assessing a wide range of moderately to highly intimate topics on a Likert-type (1–7) scale, has also been limited in its emphasis—focusing, until very recently, on overall disclosure of multiple topics rather than on disclosure of what is most relevant to specific clients.

Thus, Hill et al. (2000) as well as Kelly (2000) concluded that research with more refined methodology is needed in order to adequately investigate the relationship between disclosure and outcome. This viewpoint can hardly be overemphasized. As noted earlier, it is virtually impossible to specify the nature of the outcome–disclosure relationship without adding many other variables into the equation. To the list enumerated in the beginning of this chapter (the client's penchant for disclosure; the content, relevance, and timing of specific disclosures; the therapeutic relationship), other variables might now be added, including the patient's diagnosis, reasons for nondisclosure, the degree of emotionality contained in the disclosure, and the therapist's reaction to the disclosure. In regard to this last point, research suggests that therapists' interventions serve as powerful influences on patients' behaviors. For example, some early studies of psychotherapy (e.g., Spiesman, 1959) have indicated that when therapists' interpretations are too intense, patients' resistance increases. Analogously, therapists who are too intense (e.g., aggressively inquisitive or personally reactive) in response to their patients' disclosures are likely to inhibit further disclosures. There is also some preliminary evidence to indicate that highly disclosing therapists may facilitate greater client disclosure, at least in those cases where the client has been primed to believe that high therapist disclosure is appropriate for effective psychotherapy (Derlega, Lovell, & Chaikin, 1976). In addition, findings from a recent study of mine (Farber et al., 2004) indicate that therapists who are empathic, affirming, and nonjudgmental make patients' disclosures easier.

Other than methodological issues, what else emerges from this literature? Clearly, further research is needed to learn more about the relative effects of different types of disclosures and nondisclosures. For example, does the reluctance to reveal the details of a long-standing childhood trauma or recent marital argument (what Hill et al., 1993, deem "secrets") have the same effect on therapeutic process and outcome as the refusal to disclose immediately experienced negative feelings to one's therapist? Do disclosures that are solicited by the therapist have different properties than those that seem more spontaneously generated? In addition, more empirical work needs to be done to further test Stiles' "fever model." It may be the case, for example, that moderate levels of distress are reduced through disclosure in therapy, whereas both high and low levels are relatively immune to these benefits. Moreover, far more work needs to be done in the area of individual differences, studying the extent to which certain types of patients (categorized, for example, by diagnosis, attachment style, or sensitizer–repressor typology) experience particular consequences of disclosure and nondisclosure. For some psychotherapy patients, disclosure may reduce symptoms; for other patients, disclosure may have little impact on symptoms but may increase self-awareness and quality of interpersonal relationships; and, for still others, disclosure may have no discernible positive effects and may even cause greater distress across multiple indices.

Thus, many questions remain unanswered about the process and effects of disclosure in therapy. It would not at all be surprising if, ultimately, the question posed in this area mirrors the "specificity" question asked in contemporary psychotherapy research: "What interventions, used by which therapists, have what effects on which clients experiencing what symptoms?" In the case of disclosure, the question investigated might be: "What types of therapist interventions yield what kinds of short- and long-term positive and negative consequences in response to what types of disclosures and nondisclosures made by which clients with what therapeutic goals and levels of distress?"

Finally, the following thought may be reiterated. Although self-disclosure may be a means toward health and may be associated with therapeutic improvement, it is surely not the only means to health and surely not the only source of therapeutic benefit. In this regard, Storr (1996) relates the following anecdote:

> A patient whom I was treating . . . once lay on the couch for fifty minutes without saying anything at all. Partly out of curiousity [sic], partly out of a sense that something important was taking place, I also said nothing. The atmosphere was peaceful and happy. At the end of the session, she said that this had been the best of all our meetings so far. (p. 231)

CHAPTER 5

Multicultural Perspectives on Patient Disclosure

A man's capable of understanding anything—how the ether
vibrates, and what's going on in the sun—but how any other man
can blow his nose differently from him, that he's incapable of
understanding.

—TURGENEV (1861, p. 102)

Hai Bin, tell me—what are the two things you think about most,
that pass through your mind most, whether you like it not?' He
paused for a few seconds, scratching his head, then answered
'eating and sleeping.' I was so full of hope that our culture gap
would magically be bridged that I could not accept this.

—SALTZMAN (1990, p. 99)

Self-disclosure varies widely among patients. Previous chapters have noted
that several factors may affect disclosure patterns and the likelihood of positive outcome, including patient variables (e.g., sensitizer–repressor typology and attachment status), therapist variables (e.g., empathic responsiveness), and treatment variables (e.g., strength of alliance, length of therapy,
and therapeutic orientation). The results of studies suggest that securely
attached "sensitizers," in therapy for longer periods of time and engaged in
a strong therapeutic alliance with an affirming and nonjudgmental therapist, are likely to be highly self-disclosing of relevant personal information,
especially in the presence of a highly disclosing therapist. Results further
suggest that a patient's capacity to discuss old material in new cognitive
and/or emotional terms increases greatly the probability of deriving therapeutic benefit from disclosure.

What has been absent to this point is a consideration of the ways in which culture, especially nationality and ethnicity, might affect the process of disclosure. Let us consider several examples of how nationality influences the domain of what is and is not discussed in general conversation. Finnish people avoid small talk and accept silence for far longer periods than Americans. Their culture and language tend to limit personal affirmations and intimacies. A revealing quip is told about the Finnish man who loved his wife so much he almost told her he loved her. Similarly, in Great Britain, the principle tenaciously observed among the upper class is that one never reveals one's feelings in public (Lyall, 2005). In Sweden, too, there is great respect for personal boundaries; people simply don't ask personal questions. On the other hand, in Israel, bus riders will share personal information, give advice, and solicit opinions from others. Americans and French people also differ substantially on what can and can't be disclosed openly: "If sex is the great taboo in American life and movies, money is the subject that can shock the pants off a Frenchman. . . . Talking about your finances, even among friends and family, is considered indiscreet, tactless, vulgar, and vaguely American" (Hohenadel, 2004, p. 13). Although these examples are not in the realm of psychotherapy per se, nor based on hard research findings, they nevertheless provide some indication of how culture mediates the boundaries of disclosure.

This chapter, then, discusses patient disclosure from a multicultural perspective. Despite the paucity of empirical studies focusing on this issue, there is a fair amount of theory and sociological data that provide some understanding of cultural influences on disclosure in therapy. Following these introductory paragraphs, I move to a review of why research into multicultural issues affecting psychotherapy is both necessary and long overdue. From there, I briefly consider ethnic differences in language use and then turn to a longer discussion of how cultural differences regarding the notion of "self" impacts upon disclosure. The balance of this chapter focuses specifically on Asian, African American, and Latino patients' disclosure in Western-style therapy.

One other preliminary note: Ethnic minorities cover a diverse range of cultures and traditions. The simplest approach to defining racial/ethnic minorities is that they are groups comprised of nonwhite individuals. Nevertheless, defining racial–ethnic minority groups is complicated by the heterogeneity of racial compositions both within and across groups. Each major racial minority category in the United States, including Asians, African Americans, and Latinos, is an amalgamation of distinct national origin groups, cultures, and extensive geographic locations. According to Bradshaw (1994), the Asian culture alone represents ethnicities from China, Japan, the Philippines, Korea, India, Pakistan, Bangladesh, Southeast Asia (e.g., Vietnam, Laos, Cambodia), and the Pacific Islands (e.g., Hawaii, Melanesia, Micronesia, Polynesia). Thus, while the designation of minority status is shared by numerous ethnic groups and at times can serve as a common link between diverse cultures, the history and experience of how each minority group and subgroup has had to acculturate to the majority culture is typically distinctive.

THE IMPORTANCE OF CULTURE, THE LACK OF RESEARCH

One of the most trenchant criticisms leveled at 20th-century psychology is that it has embraced a one-size-fits-all mentality. According to this perspective, clinical theory and practice have too often ignored individual differences, especially those associated with gender, race, and culture. Relatedly, psychological theories and research have been castigated for assuming that findings based primarily or exclusively on Caucasian samples will necessarily generalize to the universe of other populations. Partly in reaction to these criticisms, partly in response to the growing numbers of minorities in U.S. society (27% according to the 1994 census report, and growing), and partly in reaction to increasing awareness and even appreciation of cultural differences, the field of psychology has begun to accept and even, at times, embrace diversity. Mental health associations now routinely adopt diversity as a conference theme, and professional organizations, including the American Psychological Association, have encouraged and even mandated practitioners and training programs to be more aware of and sensitive to multicultural issues. Multicultural competence and diversity issues are increasingly being addressed and incorporated into academic curricula and mental health services (Constantine & Gloria, 1999; Miranda, Azocar, Organista, Munoz, & Lieberman, 1996).

Still, much of the research in the field suffers from cultural myopia. Most psychotherapy research—indeed, most psychological research—relies on a narrow database disproportionately comprised of white middle-class undergraduate college populations (Miranda, 1996; Sears, 1986). Consistent with this, what we know about patient disclosure is based almost exclusively on data collected by nonminority researchers using nonminority samples of both patients and therapists. Despite Jourard's occasional inclusion of cross-cultural factors in his early research on self-disclosure in the 1960s and 1970s, subsequent empirical work has tended not to examine the relationship of race, ethnicity, or culture to self-disclosure patterns in psychotherapy. With the exception of an article comparing Caucasian and Asian American disclosure patterns in therapy (Berano & Farber, 2006), recent studies have not included sufficient numbers of minority patients to investigate racial/ethnic differences. For example, in Farber and Hall's (2002) study of patient disclosure, minority participants were significantly underrepresented: The sample consisted of 138 whites (94%), 2 blacks

(1.4%), 2 Asians (1.4%), and 5 Hispanics (3.4%). Similarly, in Kelly et al.'s (1996) study of secret keeping in therapy, 95% of the sample was white, and in Kahn et al.'s (2001) study of "distress disclosure" among undergraduate users of a campus counseling center, the authors noted that almost all of the participants were European American or Caucasian.

In addition to the lack of representation of culturally diverse participants, the research on self-disclosure in therapy suffers from another significant limitation, one related to the idea of social constructivism (e.g., Gergen, 1985). The notion here is that what we study and how and where and when and with whom we study it is inextricably linked to the culture in which we live. The assumptions made about what would or would not be discussed in therapy, the hypotheses regarding which variables might affect these tendencies, the measures chosen to represent these assumptions, the questions posed by the researchers, the methodology employed, the inclusionary and exclusionary criteria used for recruiting patients and therapists, the setting of the research, and, of course, the findings reported and conclusions reached all reflect a particular research tradition operating in a particular culture at a particular point in time.

Thus, what Marsella (1982) articulated nearly 25 years ago is still essentially true today: that empirical studies in this area seldom consider how different cultures define normality or distress, or how these conceptual differences may affect the process of disclosure in therapy. On a macro level, the interplay of traditional cultural values and belief systems (Carter, 1991), sociocultural and sociopolitical history (Comas-Diaz & Greene, 1994), and the level of embedded identity within one's cultural heritage (Blustein, 1994; Blustein & Noumair, 1996) is likely to influence the extent to which an individual reveals his or her innermost feelings and problems to a therapist. On a micro level, factors such as acculturation to the dominant culture, socioeconomic status, and the nature of one's upbringing are likely to moderate the general approach, content, and style of disclosures (Adler et al., 1994; Atkinson, Morten, & Sue, 1998; Loo, Tong, & True, 1989; Sue & Sue, 1999).

THE IMPACT OF LINGUISTIC STYLE AND NOTIONS OF "SELF" ON PATTERNS OF SELF-DISCLOSURE

The act of verbally communicating is a process inherent in all people (Mitchell, 2002), a commonality that cuts across all ethnic, racial, and cultural divides. Nevertheless, marked differences exist in the value that different racial/ethnic groups place on verbal communication and in the stylistic means through which they express information. Significant differences also exist in how different cultures view the idea of "self" and the necessity of sharing personal information. How, then, might such cultural differences play out in the realm of self-disclosure, especially in the context of a psychotherapeutic setting that is sanctioned by the dominant culture?

Western Anglo-American cultures tend to value and rely heavily on verbal language skills to express thoughts and feelings. Verbal acumen is the preferred means to provide and receive clear and direct information, and Western-oriented psychotherapies reflect this bias. However, different racial/ethnic minority groups and individuals identify and process problems in diverse verbal and nonverbal ways. For example, Asian, black, and Latino clients may use nonstandard English (e.g., Ebonics), shorter and/or incomplete sentences with less grammatical elaboration, or nonverbal cues, such as a stare or silence (Sue & Sue, 1999). This may lead to communicative and diagnostic misunderstanding on the part of the upper-middle-class Caucasian therapist who is accustomed to communication involving more standard use of grammar and syntax and less reliance on nonverbal cues (Sue & Sue, 1999). These stylistic differences may also lead to unwarranted assumptions about the extent of patient resistance and may damage, sometimes irreparably, the therapeutic alliance. Miscommunication is also likely to result from basic deficits in the language skills of those for whom English is not a first language (assuming English as the only language available for the therapist). Thus, self-disclosure of information from a minority patient to a nonminority therapist cannot proceed with the same assumptions as when both patient and therapist have similar ethnic/racial origins or identifications. The therapist must be far more alert and sensitive to potential misunderstandings based on stylistic differences in verbal expressiveness, body language, and eye contact.

Furthermore, understanding the role of self-disclosure in ethnic minority groups cannot begin by assuming that all cultures consider an individualistic sense of "self" as primary. Western European cultures tend to view the "self" as an "I" that represents an individual who is independent, autonomous, and unique (Triandis, 1988). According to Markus and Kitayama (1991), an "independent construal of self" is manifest through promoting individual goals, asserting, validating and appreciating one's internal attributes, and maintaining a bounded and separate sense of self. Conversely, an "interdependent construal of self" is more characteristic of non-Western cultures in which the "self" is part of a social network in which one's behavior is largely contingent on the feelings, thoughts, and actions of others. In other words, the interdependent self is relationally oriented and situationally driven (Yeh & Hwang, 2000). The role of an interdependent self is to promote the goals of others, act in an indirect manner, and restrain individualistic interests in order to preserve harmony within the social context (Hsu, 1981; Markus & Kitayama, 1991).

As an example of how an individual's culturally mediated sense of self can affect disclosure and the entire process of psychotherapy, consider the following statement from a female Mexican client (in Seeley, 2000):

"A lot of these issues . . . around my family, in terms of where I am fit in in [sic] the family, and my responsibilities to them [have] been hard for her [my therapist] to handle, I think. I think she got it, though, she got if after like the third time around, you know, issues of poverty. My sister's not rich, my sister's poor . . . and after the couple times of saying, 'You're not responsible for your sister,' I'm like, 'You don't know what the hell you're talking about,' she's really been able to acknowledge that there's some things that I'm just not going to change." (p. 144)

In a similar fashion, non-Western aspects of "self" can be understood by considering the complementary concepts of individualism and collectivism. Individualism emphasizes self-orientation, self-sufficiency, and personal gain. In collectivism, there is a sense of "oneness" among individuals in which sacrifice of individual goals to meet the needs and concerns of others is paramount (Triandis, 1988). For example:

In many collectivist cultures, a 15-year-old child who was not working hard in school would reflect poorly on the entire family. If the student was referred for psychotherapy, it would be to not only assist the student in improving grades, but also has implications for the larger family system. Better grades would reflect on good upbringing. . . . Therapists from individualistic cultures may erroneously focus on individual achievement and self-esteem, highlighting the personal accomplishments of the student, rather than the success of the family through the child's success. (Chung, Bemak, & Kilink, 2002, p. 122)

Thus, collectivist values might well deter individuals from disclosing information that would place another in an unfavorable position. Individualistic values would pose no such threat. It is, however, important to remember that most individuals fall at neither end of the individualistic–collectivist continuum, and thus virtually all patients in therapy struggle to find an appropriate balance between implicating others for one's problems and implicating only oneself. Still, as Toukmanian and Brouwers (1998) state, "Differences along the individualistic–collectivist continuum play a significant role in determining an individual's willingness to disclose" (p. 109). Their sense is that disclosing psychologically distressing information almost inevitably involves acknowledgment of "vulnerable or unfavorable aspects of the self or family" (pp. 109–110), a task of considerable difficulty for many individuals from collectivist-oriented Eastern cultures.

Complicating attempts to understand the nature of "self" from a cultural perspective is the fact that in the United States many people are biculturally competent. These are individuals who are able to utilize the language, coping skills, communicative modes, and predominant interpersonal style of their culture of origin as well as their current culture. More-over, they are able to move adaptively between these cultures without feel-ing confined to one specific cultural identity (Domanico, Crawford, & Wolfe, 1994; LaFromboise, Coleman, & Gerton, 1993; Ramirez, 1984; Yeh & Hwang, 2000).

The extent of individuals' malleability in this regard—how embedded they are in each culture (Blustein & Noumair, 1996)—is likely to affect the process of self-disclosure in therapy. It is not hard to imagine, for example, that at least some bicultural individuals would react to therapist questions in ways more closely identified with their traditional culture values than contemporary Western ones. Although excerpted from a nontherapeutic context, the following statement of a Chinese-Thai American college stu-dent describes well the nature of bicultural conflict:

> "I wish I could be open and just let out what is bothering me, to say what I feel and not keep it bottled inside. I'm an American so I should stand up for what I believe [but] instead, I keep quiet and let it pass because that is what I am taught. . . . I don't always agree with [Asian values] in theory but I generally use [them] in my actions." (in Uba, 1994, p. 124)

Insight into specific racial/ethnic minority cultural values, beliefs, tra-ditions, and communication styles can provide an understanding of the ways in which these groups might approach self-disclosure in therapy. What follows, then, is a discussion of certain Asian, African American, and Latino cultural values and traditions, along with ideas and hypotheses as to how these may affect the process of self-disclosure.

ASIAN PATIENTS AND SELF-DISCLOSURE

In this section, "Asian" refers to those of Japanese, Chinese, and Korean descent. The literature on Asian people and self-disclosure consistently places the constructs of self-disclosure and "self" within a context that incorporates philosophical, political, social, and religious aspects of Asian culture.

The place of self-disclosure in Asian cultures is quite different from that of Western societies (Chen, 1995; Sandhu, 1997; Yum, 1988; Zhang, Snowden, & Sue, 1998). Eastern cultures, specifically those of China, Japan, and Korea, have been heavily dominated by Confucian social phi-losophy and interdependent/collectivist values. As alluded to earlier, these systems emphasize verbal restraint (especially in regard to emotional expression), respect for silence, indirect communication between individu-als, and obedience to the hierarchical social and family structure (Ball, 1999; Chu, 1999; Sandhu, 1997; Shon & Ja, 1982; Sue & Sue, 1999). Priority is placed on the listener's sensitivity and ability to discern nonverbal "under the surface meaning."

Thus, the "problem" can be stated simply: Western psychotherapeutic approaches are typically highly dependent upon personal disclosure. Moreover, almost all Western therapeutic approaches (with the possible exception of marital and family therapy) reflect an implicit belief in the primacy of the individual. According to Toukmanian and Brouwers (1998), this set of assumptions privileges analytic, verbal, and introspective capacities and as such may well be "inappropriate and of questionable clinical value for individuals from non-Western cultures" (p. 107). Insight is not especially valued within many Eastern cultures; indeed, the mental strength to avoid unpleasant thoughts is emphasized and prized, as is the resolve to abstain from any disclosure that would shame family members (Sue & Sue, 1999; Toukmanian & Brouwers, 1998). Disclosures addressing here-and-now feelings toward one's therapist might also be especially difficult for individuals who have been taught to monitor and respect the feelings of another. We might expect, then, that when individuals with an interdependent sense of self engage in Western modes of psychotherapeutic treatment they become especially prone to "hidden reactions" (Hill et al., 1993)—that is, experiencing feelings toward the therapist that are not expressed.

Sue and Sue (1999) offer a trenchant example of how a therapist's obliviousness to non-Western values in regard to disclosure can undermine sensitive and effective treatment of an Asian client. Their case is of a 21-year-old Chinese American college student who came to therapy with academic and health-related issues and who presented as a depressed, anxious, and verbally constricted young man. One of the issues that emerged was that his parents wanted him to study engineering, a field that he did not like. The therapist suggested that the client was too dependent on his parents and needed to act more assertively toward them by more explicitly articulating his own needs. Following a difficult role play during which he was ultimately persuaded to state his true feelings toward his parents, the client became more withdrawn and guilt-ridden. According to Sue and Sue, the therapist failed to recognize not only the client's great hesitancy in implicitly criticizing his parents but also the client's attempt to be respectful toward him (the therapist) as well. It was the therapist's values—especially his belief in the need for open expression of feelings—that were being imposed on the client.

As noted above, reaching an agreement based on minimal amounts of verbal communication is considered an ideal form of interaction in traditional Asian culture; indeed, it is seen as a form of "same heartedness" (Tsujimura, 1987). Thus, it is the "act," based on the sincere mind, that is thought to create and sustain interpersonal relationships. In fact, "eloquent" individuals are often viewed as immature, less knowledgeable, and even dangerous (Chen, 1995; Fang & Wark, 1998). Not surprisingly, then, self-disclosure, loquaciousness, and reliance on verbal self-expression are not highly valued in these traditional segments of Asian society (Bradshaw, 1994).

In this regard, Yi (1995) offers a case in which the therapist misinterpreted her patient's purpose in seeking therapy. The patient, a Japanese woman in her late 20s, was having difficulties supervising a white male on her management team. Similar to the case described by Sue and Sue (1999), the therapist here construed the problem in terms of the patient's dependency, fears of separation from parents, and anxieties surrounding the possibility of eliciting others' disapproval. The patient, however, averred that she was happy with her living arrangements and enjoyed a good relationship with her parents. Yi concludes that the patient's "presenting problem of difficulty asserting herself to a subordinate male did not have to be understood only through the Western lens, that is, as a case of impaired autonomy and lack of individuation. . . . Instead [the patient], coming from a culture where interpersonal wishes and needs are honored and communicated indirectly and without explicit communication, was faced with a potentially face losing situation of having to explicitly make her wish known to her subordinate" (Yi, 1995, p. 310).

Some theorists (e.g., Hall, 1976; Miyanaga, 1991) have used a more sociological paradigm to explain differences in disclosure practices between Asian and American societies. They have suggested that in "high context cultures" such as Japan—where race, language, and cultural practices tend to be homogenous—verbal expression is often suppressed and individuals are unlikely to divulge their "true feelings" unless they know the person relatively well. By contrast, in culturally diverse "low context" cultures such as that of the United States, verbal expression is usually encouraged.

Research has tended to support these ideas. For example, Nakanishi (1987) found that Japanese college students rated low- and medium-level disclosure significantly more useful than high-disclosure dialogue. High self-disclosers were perceived to be the least competent communicators, and low self-disclosers the most competent communicators. Barnlund (1975, 1989) found that, whereas Japanese and Americans had similar patterns of preferred and avoided conversational topics—preferring conversations on "tastes and interests" and shunning conversations about finances, body-oriented, and personality issues—there were significant differences in terms of depth of disclosure. Americans disclosed significantly more on average than Japanese individuals on all topics, across all levels of intimate relationships. Chen (1995) found similar results in a study investigating differences in disclosure patterns with Chinese and American college students: Preferred conversational topics were ranked similarly by these two groups, but Americans perceived themselves as disclosing significantly more. Lastly, Asai and Barnlund (1998) explored the extent to which Japanese and Americans possess "self-knowledge" of their inner experiences and whether private and sensitive topics are disclosed to others. The authors found that Americans explored topics of religious feelings, grief, death, and positive aspects of personality and body significantly more deeply and frequently than the Japanese group.

The results of these studies suggest that Asian individuals tend to reveal less of their "private self" to others. This may pose particular difficulties in a Western mode of therapy that requires more disclosing of that which is "private" in a context that may be experienced as too "public" (or at least too nonfamilial) for Asian clients. As noted earlier, for clients imbued with a Confucian-influenced collectivist ideology, disclosure of problems and private issues to strangers is perceived as a sign of weakness that brings shame and disgrace to the family. Instead, such individuals will typically mask emotional problems, seek intrafamilial resources, or talk indirectly about problematic issues as a gesture to "save face" for the entire family (Berg & Jaya, 1993; Fang & Wark, 1998). Furthermore, because Asians tend to shun emotionally expressive individuals (Chen, 1995), highly disclosing therapists are unlikely to elicit reciprocally high degrees of disclosure from their Asian clients.

Given these differences, how do Asian clients tend to behave in therapy? According to several authors, many Asian patients view therapists as "authority figures" and "experts" and have minimal interest in exploring inner feelings, understanding the root of their problems, and obtaining insight (Berg & Jaya, 1993; Fang & Wark, 1998; Shonfeld-Ringel, 2001; Sue & Sue, 1999; Yi, 1995). Yi suggests that Asian patients may view their therapist as someone who provides guidance and advice on issues concerning work, education, time management, or career-related dilemmas. And Berg and Jaya (1993) advise therapists working with Asian patients that brief contact focusing on crises intervention or immediate problem solving may be especially consistent with Asian patients' expectations. Others (e.g., Bachelor, 1995; Ham, 1993; Shonfeld-Ringel, 2001) have suggested that a particular form of empathy, one that strives for a holistic awareness of harmony between individuals, is a crucial component of culturally sensitive treatment with Asian clients.

The literature also suggests that when focal psychoeducational strategies are utilized in the context of a highly empathic, culture-specific therapy, Asian clients continue treatment for longer periods of time and are willing to explore deeper relational issues (Tang, 1997; Tung, 1991). Berg and Jaya's (1993) presentation of the case of Mrs. Kim, a 67-year-old Korean woman, illustrates many of these issues. This apparently depressed client had attempted suicide by slitting her throat with a butcher knife. Mrs. Kim had felt humiliated for being placed with her husband in an elderly housing project by her son due to her cultural clashes with her son's children. She felt she had failed as a mother. In treatment, Mrs. Kim was able to self-disclose and open up after the therapist reframed her son's behavior as misguided but also as a gesture of responsibility to his children, which to a large extent reflected the cultural values he had learned from Mrs. Kim. At a 1-year follow-up, Mrs. Kim was doing well and there was no recurrence of depression.

The research and theory presented in this section point consistently to cultural differences that would lead us to conclude that Asian clients are likely to struggle with personal disclosures to their therapists. However, Asian American clients might well act in ways that are contrary to these findings, especially if they are relatively acculturated to Western customs and interpersonal styles or relatively aware of the demand characteristics of Western-style therapies. In fact, research indicates that acculturation plays a significant role in help-seeking attitudes for Asians (Atkinson & Gim, 1989), so that more acculturated clients may struggle less with self-disclosure. Furthermore, a recent study found that a heterogeneous sample of Asian American therapy patients disclosed to the same extent as a comparative sample of Caucasian American patients (Berano & Farber, 2006). Clearly, though, more empirical studies are needed to evaluate the role that culture plays in the therapeutic process for Asian clients.

AFRICAN AMERICAN CLIENTS
AND SELF-DISCLOSURE

There are few empirical studies on self-disclosure and African American clients in the context of therapy. However, there is an extensive clinical literature on race and psychotherapy, at least some of which has implications for the issue of disclosure. Indeed, issues of race, racism, oppression, and cultural mistrust are recurrent themes in the literature on African Americans and psychotherapy (Greene, 1994; Ridley, 1984; Sue & Sue, 1999; Thompson, Neighbors, Munday, & Jackson, 1996).

The historical legacy of African Americans poses a unique set of challenges for the potential client in treatment and the mental health field as a whole. According to some authors (e.g., Grier & Cobbs, 1968; Sue & Sue, 1999; Vontress, 1971), depictions of white people and the predominant social system as oppressive unless proven otherwise have been necessary for the survival of African Americans within American society. From this perspective, African Americans are justifiably reluctant to expose their internal psychological world for fear of potential harm and mistreatment. This attitude is said to reflect a "healthy cultural paranoia" (Grier & Cobbs, 1968; Ridley, 1984) or "paranorm" (Sue & Sue, 1999) and may be viewed as an adaptive rather than dysfunctional coping mechanism. Therefore, the degree to which an African American client has experienced and continues to experience racism, oppression, and cultural mistrust may significantly influence the way he or she initially approaches and subsequently deals with issues of disclosure in therapy. As Sue and Sue (1999) note, the extent to which minorities self-disclose in therapy is largely dependent on their perceptions of therapists' trustworthiness, since mental health professionals are often viewed as extensions or agents of "the establishment."

A recent study by Sanders Thompson, Bazile, and Akbar (2004) confirmed some of these hypotheses. The authors conducted a qualitative study of African American consumers of mental health services as well as of their family and community members with no prior history of treatment. They found that "issues of trust" were a significant concern for these participants. That is, although participants acknowledged that psychotherapy could be helpful, they were nevertheless not convinced, nor trusted, that therapists possessed sufficient knowledge and understanding of African American life and hardships. Moreover, these participants wondered whether therapists continue to hold stereotypes of minorities. One respondent held the following view of psychologists: "It doesn't seem like they're truly concerned about you, what you could be possibly going through. You know it's just like, 'I'm about to get paid . . . your hour is up'" (p. 23). Another participant commented directly on the relationship of trust to disclosure: "You might not trust White people. You're not going to sit and talk to somebody if you don't trust them" (p. 23).

Studies by Terrell and colleagues (Terrell & Terrell, 1984; Watkins & Terrell, 1988) have shown that client trust of therapists is a significant predictor of premature termination of therapy for African Americans. The actual relationship between these variables is complex, however: African Americans who are highly mistrustful tend to terminate counseling prematurely regardless of counselor race more than those with lower levels of mistrust. This finding, according to the authors, stems from highly mistrustful black clients' perceiving black counselors as conforming to Eurocentric views. Whereas it is important to note that these studies were conducted in another era—one usually regarded as more racially divisive—it is also certainly the case that issues of racial trust have not entirely dissipated in our society (or any other) and that they continue to play out in the context of psychotherapy in both racially mixed and racially similar dyads.

In fact, there are mixed findings regarding the effects of client–counselor racial dissimilarity. Some studies and clinical reports indicate that black clients tend to experience low levels of rapport with white therapists (Atkinson et al., 1996) and disclose less or censor more personal information to a white therapist (Plasky & Lorion, 1984; Ridley, 1984; Sue & Sue, 1999; Thompson, Worthington, & Atkinson, 1994). Ponterotto, Alexander, and Hinkston (1988) found that "similar ethnicity" was the second of 15 preferred counselor characteristics among African Americans. However, other research (Poston, Craine, & Atkinson, 1991; Thompson et al., 1994) indicates that racially mixed or black client–white counselor dyads are a concern for some clients but not others.

Here is a case example, taken from Walker (1999), in which issues arising in a racially similar dyad affected the client's level of trust and willingness to disclose:

> A first-year female law school student from the Virgin Islands was referred to therapy by her professors, who saw her "as brittle and ingratiating." When she came to her therapist's office, she professed to have no goals other than to use the time as a resource to further her academic career. The therapist, noting "subtle political undertones" to their exchanges, initiated discussions of how racial, ethnic, and hierarchical power considerations affected their relationship. Both became aware that significant ethnic and class differences stood in contrast to their racial commonality. But the real complication resided in the fact that they were two black women attempting to negotiate a relationship within the context of a white patriarchal organization. According to the therapist,
>
>> to the extent that [my patient] constructed psychological therapy as a "White" enterprise, my role as an African-American therapist was somewhat suspect. In addition, to the extent that I was a member of a socially devalued group, the therapy that I might offer was somewhat suspect. . . . At this and various other points throughout our work together, the pressing question was could I be trusted to be "real." (pp. 54–55)

Several investigators have used the modified Jourard Self-Disclosure Questionnaire (JSDQ) to analyze disclosure patterns among African Americans outside of therapy. Noel and Smith (1996), for example, evaluated the influence of student and faculty ethnicity on student willingness to disclose. The authors reported that students were more willing to disclose to faculty of the same ethnicity than to an out-group faculty member. Additional results showed that black students were reluctant to disclose to out-group faculty about racial, academic, and "sensitive" topics—findings the authors attributed to black students' fears that white faculty members would not be able to understand them or might debase their cultural beliefs, traditions, and values. Would the results of this campus study generalize to a psychotherapeutic setting? Although it is tempting to imagine that the same dynamics would play out in therapy, it is also possible that moderate to intense psychological distress (of a magnitude beyond what was studied in this investigation) would provide an impetus for self-disclosure that would either transcend racial factors or mitigate its influence.

African Americans are underrepresented in the mental health professions, so there is a strong likelihood that African American clients will work with a therapist of a different race than their own (Holzer, Goldsmith, & Ciarlo, 1998). As noted earlier, there are significant variations in the experiences of those who work with therapists of a different race. Still, because issues of trust and open disclosure are likely to be more salient in this situation than in same-race dyads, certain fundamental elements of rapport building and inquiry have been suggested. These include discussing the client's reaction to having a counselor of a different background, assessing feelings and attitudes toward therapy, determining the client's experiences with discrimination and racism, assessing positive assets of the client, and addressing external factors that may be contributing to the presenting problems (Sue & Sue, 1999).

Poston et al. (1991) coined the phrase "dissimilarity confrontation" to describe the process by which therapists attempt to facilitate cross-racial therapeutic work by openly discussing the racial, ethnic, and cultural differences between themselves and their clients. And Constantine and Kwan (2003) have noted how a combination of therapist disclosure and open discussion of racial differences can further client disclosure. Here is an example they present—specifically, of a white therapist beginning to engage in this type of process with her black client:

> Jessica (pseudonym) was a 20 year-old, Black female junior . . . at a large, predominantly White, West-coast state university. . . . She presented for psychotherapy to address feelings of lethargy, lack of motivation, anxiety, social isolation, and racial and gender discrimination. Jessica requested a female psychotherapist and was assigned a White female therapist by the agency. . . . Early in her therapy sessions, she stated that Blacks and Whites tended to think and communicate "differently" and that "we're just different." She often made such statements followed by uncharacteristically long pauses. Sensing that she hesitated to describe her frustrations further with her therapist, Jessica was asked directly how she felt about discussing her feelings and perspectives with a non-Black therapist. Jessica appeared surprised by this question and stated that she expected her therapist to listen to her without "really getting it." She also reported that she had been hesitant to discuss or elaborate on this issue because of the therapist's race.
>
> Jessica then asked her therapist whether she personally had ever been discriminated against. Her psychotherapist, who had experienced similar sexist treatment in her graduate program nearly 30 years ago, felt torn about how to answer. In response to Jessica's question, the therapist stated, "I know that feeling discriminated against must be difficult for you." Jessica became frustrated by her therapist's response and stated, "I asked you that question because I wanted to know if you really understand how I feel. Based on your response, I don't know that you do, so I'm not sure I can trust telling you more at this point." Jessica's therapist considered the pros and cons of directly answering Jessica's question and then stated, "I'm sorry I was evasive. I knew what you were needing from me at

the time you asked that question, but I guess I didn't want my response to deter you from your own issues and progress. I would have to honestly report that I also have experienced sexism and it is painful. However, an additional element you're currently experiencing is racism, and I'm wondering how you're feeling about having to deal with these two issues concurrently?" (pp. 585–586)

Do these ideas "work"? In a study by Poston et al. (1991), dissimilarity confrontation and willingness to self-disclose were positively correlated, although that relationship was not statistically significant. Additional findings of the same study suggest that African Americans disclose more to a white therapist as their income increases, and that disclosure decreases with more education. The authors speculated that increases in income bring more exposure to a predominantly white working world for the black client, which leads to more rapport and trust building with Whites. However, the investigators also suggested that more education leads to more knowledge of racial oppression, which results in less disclosure to a white therapist.

Consistent with the ideas of those espousing the importance of explicitly addressing racial issues in cross-racial therapeutic dyads, Sanders Thompson et al. (2004) found that client self-disclosure was enhanced when counselors focused on racial and cultural concerns specific to the African American client rather than on general issues unrelated to culture. About one-third of the therapy clients in this study believed that if race was not discussed in a therapeutic relationship, it was due to the therapist's racism or discomfort. Another third averred that they would be relieved and would welcome the opportunity to speak honestly if their therapist initiated such a discussion. Many commented that they did not bring up some clinically relevant material, including "experiences with racism, discrimination, the stress of 'paying bills,' balancing work and family life, and exposure to community trauma," because of their apprehension that the therapist would not understand these situations.

In sum, studies of African Americans and disclosure vary considerably in regard to methodology and focus. Most importantly, and unfortunately, few studies have focused explicitly on actual disclosure in therapy, leaving much to learn about the dynamics of this process as it unfolds among African American clients.

LATINOS AND SELF-DISCLOSURE

The term "Latino" is used herein for its gender inclusiveness and as a reflection of political, economic, and geographic accuracy of representation (Chapa & Valencia, 1993; Falicov, 1998). Latinos of America represent a unique mosaic of historical, political, cultural, and geographical differences. However, despite myriad subgroups, the common language of Spanish is shared by all, often (though not always) facilitating an affinity among Latino people. For the most part, Latinos in this discussion refer to those of Mexican, Puerto Rican, and Cuban ancestry, the most common ethnic subgroups represented in the psychotherapy and self-disclosure literatures (Falicov, 1998; Rogler, Malgady, & Rodriguez, 1989; Snell, Miller, Belk, Garcia-Falconi, & Hernandez-Sanchez, 1989; Sue & Sue, 1999).

As was true of Asian and African Americans, empirical research focused on self-disclosure among Latino clients in therapy is essentially nonexistent. Therefore, much of the present discussion relies on extrapolations from analogue studies (primarily of college students), sociological observations, and clinical case reports.

The cultural traditions of Latinos are rooted in collectivism, strong and extended family ties, patriarchal and generational hierarchies, and religious and spiritual practices (Falicov, 1998; Sabogal, Marin, Otero-Sabogal, Marin, & Perez-Stable, 1987; Sue & Sue, 1999; Vasquez, 1994). The cumulative impact of these traditions is such that exercising one's individuality or autonomy is uncommon. Indeed, "familismo" cannot be overestimated as an integral part of Latino culture, for it defines the inclusiveness, constant involvement, and rich connections among Latino family members that can span several generations (Falicov, 1998; Lopez & Guarnaccia, 2000). Roland (1994) coined the term "familial self" to describe the process of incorporating the importance of close relationships within one's sense of self while maintaining an inner reserve of unshared feelings, or "private self."

"Respeto" (respect) is another aspect of the Latino family hierarchy that affects interpersonal relations and self-expression (Falicov, 1998). The unquestioned authority of parents is typically what organizes and controls all forms of self-expression of children, and subsequently of adults as well. "Simpatia," a derivative and outward display of respeto, encourages harmony and avoidance of interpersonal conflicts through emphases on politeness, compliments, friendliness, patient explanations (e.g., by "talking nicely"), and, most importantly in regard to self-disclosure, indirect, implicit, and covert communication (Falicov, 1998; Triandis, Lisansky, Marin, & Bentancourt, 1984). Alvarez (1999) presents a good illustration of many of these themes:

> Sonia, age 35, came from the Dominican Republic as an international student. . . . [She] sought therapy because of anxiety attacks and difficulties with sleeping and concentration. She also felt depressed and unclear about what might be precipitating her symptoms. . . . In Sonia's family, direct emotional expression was considered a weakness and associated with shame. Communication was usually superficial. . . . This seemed to under-

lie her difficulty with revealing her symptoms during the initial stage of psychotherapy. . . . She felt anxious about having her vulnerabilities explored and ashamed of allowing anyone to be privy to her sadness, a feeling which represented a loss of control. (pp. 107–109)

As noted above, few empirical studies have focused on Latino disclosure in therapy. The one notable exception is Snell et al.'s (1989) analogue study that investigated gender and cultural differences in disclosing eight positive and negative emotions (depression, jealous, anxiety, anger, happiness, calmness, fear, apathy) to male and female friends and therapists. The authors found that Mexican females report significantly greater emotional disclosures to female and male therapists on all topics, with the exception of fear and apathy to male therapists. However, these results must be interpreted with caution, since the findings were based on retrospective self-reports and no attempts were made to verify whether any of the participants actually had therapists.

Three studies in the 1980s (Franco, Malloy, Gonzalez, 1984; LeVine & Franco, 1981; Molina & Franco, 1986) used Jourard's disclosure inventory (JSDQ) to investigate general disclosure patterns among whites and Mexican Americans/Latinos. Findings were mixed. In LeVine and Franco's study, white females reported the highest disclosures, followed by Latinas, white males, and Latino males. This finding corroborated Littlefield's (1974) earlier work on this topic. In contrast, Molina and Franco found mean disclosure scores were greatest for white males, followed by Mexican American females, white females, and Mexican American males. Latinas seem to disclose significantly more than Latinos (Franco et al., 1984; LeVine & Franco, 1981; Molina & Franco, 1986), perhaps because Latina immigrant mothers are especially inclined toward encouraging their daughters to become "Americanized" (Akamatsu, 1995; Falicov, 1998). Another explanation for findings that Latinas disclose more than Latinos can be found in the concept of "machismo": the attitude that Latino men are expected to embody, characterized by displays of virility, physical strength, denial of vulnerability, and, most salient in this regard, the ability to suffer in silence (Falicov, 1998). However, the following case study clearly indicates that Latino men will disclose their feelings, especially if they are of a serious nature, within the boundaries of a safe and ethnically sensitive therapeutic setting. The case is of a Latino man who was beset with suicidal depression and anxiety:

He could not talk to his relatives and friends . . . because they would think he was crazy. The therapist he had would not ask him questions because she wanted him to talk without being asked. But he could not express his feelings without being asked. The community mental health center he attended allowed him to change therapists. The new therapist asked him questions and he expressed his sadness. To improve his therapy, Mr. Rios brought to his new therapist two cassettes of tangos because it was important for her to understand the kind of music which fit his nostalgic feelings. (Rogler et al., 1989, p. 99)

Findings are inconsistent as to whether ethnically similar dyads facilitate or inhibit disclosures by Latinos. For example, LeVine and Franco (1981) found that Latino male disclosures were equal to those of white male, white female, and Latina participants when a Latina was the recipient of disclosures. And Noel and Smith (1996) found that Latino college students' level of disclosure was significantly higher to in-group (e.g., ethnically similar) than to out-group faculty. Furthermore, Latinos disclosed the least to "out-group" (e.g., ethnically dissimilar) faculty members in comparison to their White and African American peers. These results confirm Sue and Sue's (1999) contention regarding ethnic minority preference for racially similar therapeutic dyads.

On the other hand, Franco et al. (1984) found that patterns of high self-disclosure were associated with a cross-ethnic mix. Latinos disclosed more to Anglo-American research administrators, and Anglo-Americans disclosed more to Latino administrators. Acosta and Sheehan (1978) found similar results in an analogue study in which Mexican American college students were less willing to disclose to a Mexican American therapist. It is difficult to reconcile these results with the studies described above. One possibility, though, is that the samples that preferred racially similar counselors were less proficient in English. Bilingual patients often have difficulty expressing emotions in a second language, and patients (or participants in studies) may be aware of the potential confusion involved in switching between languages in order to make oneself understood. In this regard, too, there is some literature to suggest that, for some Latino clients, speaking English serves as a protective "shield" in that it allows them to distance themselves from potentially shameful clinically sensitive material (Seeley, 2000).

To the extent, though, that there is some dynamic that serves to make cross-racial disclosures easier, the explanation may lie in the nature of Latino family pride. That is, influenced by this cultural characteristic, Latino individuals may strive to keep negative perceptions of themselves or their family from ethnically similar individuals. Seeley (2000) provides an example:

Maria found that being in treatment with an Anglo therapist . . . afforded her novel opportunities. For example, she was able to explore painful childhood material and issues related to her experiences as an outsider in the university community—issues that she had found impossible to discuss with her family—with her psychotherapist. Maria also assumed that an

Anglo therapist would be more likely than a Latina therapist to maintain the confidentiality of her disclosures. "I was very uncomfortable with the idea of taking my issues to a Latino in this area, because it's so confined." (p. 143)

There is insufficient evidence to judge whether therapist self-disclosure facilitates disclosure among Latino clients. The one investigation of this topic (Cherbosque, 1987) was an analogue study in which Mexican students disclosed more than Americans and viewed counselors who refrained from self-disclosure as more expert, professional, and trustworthy than did American students. Both Mexican and American students reported that they would be most willing to disclose to a counselor who did not personally self-disclose, especially during the early phases of therapy. No conclusions should be drawn from a single study; moreover, there is some clinical evidence to suggest that therapist disclosure can be helpful to a Latino client struggling to articulate his or her experiences. Here (Falicov, 1998), the therapist's disclosure seems to help a client get in touch with and process emotions connected with her own migration experience:

> I remember one of my first therapy clients, a newly married young woman who had come from Puerto Rico to accompany her husband. . . . She was very depressed and missed her home and her country very much. She kept repeating that it was like starting all over again, having to learn everything from scratch. . . . I felt her pain as we explored details. I told her that for me too, when I first came to this country, it was so much like starting all over again. Even simple behaviors were no longer automatic. . . . As I relayed these anecdotes to my client, she cried for a long time. . . . Later she told me that the memories of that session made a difference for her. She felt she had received permission to feel her feelings. (pp. 52–53)

Thus, there are multiple dimensions of cultural overlay that affect the self-disclosure patterns of Latinos. Furthermore, there are numerous inconsistencies in the literature on this issue. Studies are needed that incorporate sophisticated assessments of acculturation levels and racial identity of a demographically diverse group of Latino psychotherapy patients. In addition, studies employing qualitative methodology, specifically tailored to Latino culture and Latino experiences in therapy, would serve to advance our understanding of the particular dynamics of Latino disclosure in therapy.

SUMMARY

Many Asian, African American, and Latino individuals maintain a degree or style of interpersonal communication that is not in accord with the expectations or practices of Anglo-European individuals in Western societies. For members of these minority groups, less personal disclosure "makes sense" as a response to an oppressive sociopolitical history and experience, as a reflection of revered philosophical and spiritual traditions, and as a means to reduce disagreements and promote harmony among others. Thus, concealment may be perceived as culturally respectful and purposeful. On the other hand, these cultural traditions may make it difficult for individuals to realize the potential salutary benefits of interpersonal disclosure. In addition, cultural differences in self-disclosure may not be well understood by some therapists, especially older therapists who received their education before the advent of multicultural training.

In most Westernized forms of therapy, the tendency to conceal is typically seen as counterproductive, a manifestation of resistance. Not surprisingly, then, as therapists and patients from diverse groups increasingly interact, complex and problematic interactions may arise that are clearly neither the "fault" of minority clients nor Western-oriented therapy providers. Each group has strong and culturally bound perceptions of psychological problems and the appropriate means to overcome them. Hence, to pathologize a reluctance to disclose, as Jourard (1971b) essentially did, reflects (in contemporary hindsight) a culturally myopic assessment of clients whose backgrounds and value reflect a very different set of beliefs about the primacy of individual needs. But, of course, such misperceptions continue to occur. Toukmanian and Brouwers (1998) offer the example of a white middle-class therapist who, unaware of others' values and norms, misconstrues and reacts insensitively to an Asian client's relative lack of disclosure in therapy. Their professed hope is that "increased awareness could lead the therapist to understand that the client's reticence [to disclose] may be a reflection of the "constraints' of culture" (p. 118).

As noted earlier, there are significant methodological limitations of the studies reviewed here. Findings in this area tend to be based on analogue studies, self-reports, and simulated counseling interviews, all done with a disproportionately high number of white college undergraduates. Ideally, studies would be based on actual clients in therapy, of multiple ages, and of Asian, African American, and Latino descent. Moreover, the current instruments used to measure disclosure tend either to be outdated or to include topics and questions that may not be culturally relevant to the respondent. Thus, actual disclosure among minority patients in therapy may yield results distinct from the findings of the extant research.

Although the research is "soft," it would be hard to argue with the need expressed in the literature for clinical sensitivity to disclosure modes that are mediated by cultural considerations. Clinicians should be aware that multiple factors may influence disclosure and that some important disclosures may be offered nonverbally. Thus, when working with clients from racial/ethnic backgrounds different from their own, therapists need to consider not only these individuals' language skills (e.g., fluency in English) and preferred communicative style (e.g., vocal tone and inflection, body language, and eye contact) but also their degree of acculturation, the extent to which they value emotional expressiveness, their level of adherence to religious and spiritual beliefs, their migration and relocation experiences, and their family structure and level of education (Carter, 1991; Falicov, 1998; Hui & Triandis, 1986; Sue & Sue, 1999). Therapeutic sensitivity to these issues—which would also include explicit discussion of racial/ethnic differences, the solidity of the relationship, and how well one is hearing what needs to be heard—is likely not only to facilitate patient disclosure of salient therapeutic material but also to increase mutual satisfaction with the process and outcome of therapy.

CHAPTER 6

Historical Perspectives on Therapist Disclosure

We are all rather transparent to those who want to see.
—SINGER (1977, p. 191)

Should it be only the patient who self discloses? What might happen if therapists were to reveal themselves more extensively?
—YALOM (1999, p. 253)

I tell a client that I too feel angry when I hear stories about his abuse; I share with a client that I, too, have had a car stolen and how violated I felt; I express to a client that, while I fear that the word may be experienced by her as patronizing, I nevertheless feel "proud" of her; I acknowledge to a client that I, too, feel frustrated by how stuck our work sometimes gets, though I still believe strongly that we will find a way; I respond to a client's direct query and let her know where I will be going on vacation, and I let her know that I will miss her as well; in response to a question, I offer that I didn't particularly like some recent movie; I let a client know that I too have been injured playing basketball and that it affected me both physically and psychologically; I tell a client that it would affect me profoundly if she were, in fact, to commit suicide and that I do worry about this possibility; I agree to give reprints of a recent article of mine to an interested client; in response to a client's question, I offer some basic information about a religious ceremony that the client wishes to know more about; "yes," I say to a client, I too have lost a father to a slow death, and I know it hurts deeply; I recommend my favorite Chinese restaurant to a couple wishing to go out to eat after a session; I am aware of how most of my clients who come to sessions at my home have, on occasion, met my wife in the driveway, seen my children riding bikes in the street, or been sniffed by my dog when she finds her way downstairs to the office.

Clearly, these responses cover a vast territory. Some reflect a part of me that only rarely emerges in therapy; some are quite consistent with my usual way of being with clients. Some responses were elicited by patients, whereas others were spontaneous reactions to their feelings or behaviors. Some responses were essentially factual, others primarily emotional. Some were more revealing of a private aspect of my life, whereas other statements, though necessarily mediated by my own style and dynamics, were more reflective of my professional role. Some were in the service of offering support, others in the service of offering advice, and still others were offered in the hope of normalizing experiences perceived by the client as aberrant. However, these statements, while accurate, are also somewhat post hoc rationalizations for behaviors that seemed simply to be in the service of more genuine and helpful engagement with a particular client at a particular moment.

All the responses noted above have, at one time or another, been considered by some theorists as falling under the rubric of therapist disclosure. On the other hand, some theorists would allow that only one or two of these examples truly belong in the set entitled to be called therapist disclosures. There are strong differences in opinion regarding definition and, relatedly, passionate arguments about the appropriate clinical use of disclosures. Indeed, the lack of a consensual definition for what constitutes therapist disclosure has muddied clinical discussions of its benefits and drawbacks and has also impeded the advancement of both theory and research in the area. A large part of the problem here is that therapist disclosures tend to fall on the boundary between personal and professional behavior.

A history of the ways in which therapist disclosure has been viewed by prominent therapists across several orientations may provide a useful context for discussion in subsequent chapters of related clinical and research issues. We may begin by referencing what was noted in Chapters 1 and 2—that contemporary interest in the issue of therapist disclosure is a phenomenon attributable in great measure to a significant paradigm shift within the declining but still influential psychoanalytic community. Over the past few decades, psychodynamically oriented therapy in virtually all its myriad forms has become more interpersonally oriented, that is, more focused on the interactions between therapist and patient and on what can be learned from such exchanges. In therapies that are more "relational," therapist abstinence and anonymity are no longer viewed as especially desirable or helpful qualities. Instead, the therapist is exhorted to be active, engaged, empathic, and genuine in expressing his or her feelings regarding the process and content of what is unfolding in the room. Therapist openness and disclosure are integral aspects of this newer healing paradigm.

Perhaps as an indirect result of these developments, or perhaps as a consequence of its own natural development, cognitive-behavioral therapy (CBT)—arguably the most popular form of therapy currently practiced in this country—has also become more relationally oriented and its practitioners more disclosing. Robert Leahy, a prominent member of the CBT community, stated the following: "It is important to recognize that what most therapists are doing when they are doing cognitive-behavioral therapy is *not* cognitive-behavioral therapy; rather, they are relating to another person" (2001, p. 259, emphasis in original). Could even experienced therapists accurately determine the theoretical orientation of the therapist in the following transcript?

> THERAPIST: You know when you've been saying that you're the sickest person I've ever seen, I think I haven't been hearing you the way you need to be heard.
> PATIENT: What do you mean?
> THERAPIST: I've been trying to convince you that you have a lot of good qualities—I've been acting like a cheerleader.
> PATIENT: You don't understand how bad I feel.
> THERAPIST: That's very true. I've tried to think about how bad you feel. I've tried to think about the worst sadness that you have. And I think that you're right. It's impossible for me to understand how bad it is for you. I've never felt anything like the way you feel. I can only imagine that it is terrible, but I don't know what the feeling is like.

This, too, is a quote from Leahy's book *Overcoming Resistance in Cognitive Therapy* (2001, p. 77) and reflects several phenomena: the difficulty in determining the theoretical orientation of a therapist by examining portions of his or her clinical transcripts; relatedly, the extensive degree of clinical overlap even among therapists of diverse theoretical orientations (Norcross & Goldfried, 1992); and, most germane to this discussion, the extent to which therapist disclosure of feelings and discussion of clinical process now occurs even in those therapies whose origins and traditions would make one assume otherwise. In other words, therapist disclosure, in one form or another, has become a common, widely accepted aspect of quite disparate therapeutic orientations.

If these developments in psychodynamically oriented and cognitive-behavioral therapies sound vaguely familiar and not entirely revolutionary, it is because they reflect the essential tenets of humanistic therapy, most clearly articulated by Rogers in his classic 1957 paper on the "necessary and sufficient conditions" of therapeutic change. To a great extent, recent developments in contemporary psychotherapies are only "new" within rather closed therapeutic systems. Client-centered and other forms of humanistic and existential therapy had by the late 1950s adopted practices regarding therapist openness, genuineness, empathy, and disclosure that are remarkably similar to those formulated by analytic "innovators" 30 and 40 years later.

I suspect that, if he were alive today, Rogers would be perplexed and perhaps also a bit perturbed by this. The paradox that he might find unsettling is that his concepts, especially those emphasizing the healing powers of an open and genuine therapeutic relationship, are in many ways more accepted than ever by a remarkably wide variety of psychotherapists. However, at the same time, these ideas are essentially unacknowledged as originating with him or in the tradition of humanistic and client-centered therapy. It is remarkable, for example, that the late Stephen Mitchell, a brilliant and well-read scholar and one who is often given substantial credit for transforming a worn-out classical psychoanalytic institution into a revitalized relational psychodynamic movement, could write a book entitled *Relationality* (2000)—a treatise on the nature and importance of interpersonal concepts in psychotherapy—and not cite Rogers a single time.

Sadly, though, this is not surprising. Rogers was essentially dismissed by the analytic community as a "lightweight"; his clinical tenets were seen as superficial, and few in the analytic community seemed willing to take his ideas seriously, much less be influenced by them (Farber et al., 1996). And, whereas it is important to note that the new analytic vision of openness and mutuality is not synonymous with that articulated by Rogers in the late 1950s—transference is still an essential aspect of psychoanalytic practice, and contemporary analysts are far more interested than client-centered therapists in identifying the dynamics within the therapeutic relationship in order to modify recurrent dysfunctional patterns in clients' relationships—it is also clear that current ideas within the analytic community regarding the benignly influential power of an open and interactive therapeutic system were largely articulated by Rogers and his followers several decades ago. Moreover, it is likely that, well before the relational psychodynamic literature adopted a new metapsychology (discarding the major tenets of drive theory) and began affirming the benefits of a more open and mutually influential therapeutic situation, a good many analytically oriented practitioners had already been practicing therapy in ways that reflected the advantages of this approach and the unacknowledged influence of humanistic ideas.

Although I am aware of the maxim that "the plural of anecdote is not data," it still feels reasonable to presume that many analysts for many years have been far more kind, supportive, empathic, relational, and self-disclosing than the analytic literature would begin to suggest. In other words, the practice of disclosure has probably always exceeded the disclosure of this practice. Indeed, one of the great historical shortcomings of psychoanalytic psychology is the extent to which practice and theory have been divergent. It is, of course, also likely that many client-centered or humanistic therapists are more interested in the origins and dynamics of their clients' pathology than they have acknowledged. Most therapists are far more eclectic in practice than they are in their own writings or clinical presentations. Many contemporary analysts, then, act very much like Rogerians in their respect for the healing powers of being genuine, self-disclosing, and affirming to their patients. Their theoretical rationale for disclosures are often "couched" in a different metapsychological language, but the behaviors themselves would almost surely be indistinguishable based on transcripts of actual sessions.

Nevertheless, because the psychoanalytic community is considerably more influential than its humanistic/existential counterpart—with far more practitioners, professional journals, graduate schools, and postdoctoral training programs reflecting its orientation—it was not until psychoanalytically oriented clinicians began to openly incorporate and endorse this seemingly new, more relational, more disclosing approach that it became a more accepted part of the greater psychotherapeutic scene.

CULTURE AND THE CHANGING NATURE OF PSYCHOTHERAPY

Whatever the influence of one psychological tradition on others, it is clear that changes in the greater culture affect the social sciences, including the values and behavior of the participants in therapy. And although it is impossible to determine with any precision or certainty which, and to what extent, social changes contribute to shifts in clinical practice, it is likely, as noted earlier, that increased public interest over the past few decades in understanding and promoting healthy personal relationships has seeped into the general psychotherapeutic culture and at least indirectly contributed to a therapeutic climate in which some personal disclosure on the part of the therapist is an expected aspect of the relationship. Far fewer clients than ever would either expect or tolerate their therapist's adoption of an unvarying, seemingly distant, professional stance.

Other cultural forces also need to be considered in thinking about why psychotherapy, including the behavior and verbal patterns of its participants, has changed in some fundamental ways over the past 30 or 40 years. For one, the women's movement has had a major impact on the ways in which we think about psychotherapy. Beginning roughly in the mid-1960s women began to imagine job possibilities that theretofore had been impossible to consider seriously. Women who previously would have restricted their career choices to teaching, social work, or nursing began entering in far greater numbers the fields of medicine, law, and psychology. Partly as a result of the influx of women into the field, psychotherapy became distinctly more relational and therapists became distinctly more open.

There are numerous other factors that help explain why many forms of therapy have become more relationally oriented since the late 1960s—including the seminal theoretical and research contributions of such notable figures as Stephen Mitchell, Otto Kernberg, Heinz Kohut, Margaret Mahler, John Bowlby, Jessica Benjamin, and Daniel Stern—but these factors must be understood in the context of a psychotherapeutic community that was rapidly changing its gender proportions, moving in the course of a 20-year span (1970–1990) from two-thirds male to two-thirds female. If one believes that there is a fundamental tendency for women to act more "relationally" and men more "autonomously"—and there is good evidence to believe so—then theories emphasizing interdependence, relatedness, attachment, and the fundamental importance of early relationships, and therapies emphasizing mutuality, goodness of fit, genuineness, interpersonal engagement, and disclosure will be more likely to be received positively by a profession comprised primarily of women serving clients who are primarily women. It is also important to note that most men in the profession have gone along willingly, even enthusiastically, on this new path.

One small but interesting indication of the shift in psychotherapy can be observed by comparing two books—both best-selling first-person accounts of psychotherapy cases—that were written in different generations. In Robert Lindner's *The 50-Minute Hour* (1955), the author's expertise is rooted in his interpretations and his meticulous reconstructions of the origins of his patients' symptoms. By contrast, in Irvin Yalom's (1999) work *Momma and the Meaning of Life* (and also in his earlier book *Love's Executioner* [1989]), the positive outcomes noted are attributed almost exclusively to the therapist's genuineness, including his constant attempts to monitor and close the interpersonal distance between him and his patients. Indeed, in the Afterword to *Momma*, Yalom writes: "If we hold that the ideal therapeutic relationship is one of genuineness and authenticity, then shouldn't the therapist be a real person in the therapy process? As real in the therapy hour as outside of it?" (p. 253).

Furthermore, studies during the past 30 years or so have convincingly established the empirical basis of a relational approach. That is, investigations of factors that contribute to therapeutic success have consistently found that the therapeutic relationship (or "alliance") plays a significant role in positive outcomes (Horvath & Bedi, 2002). There is a strong correlation between patients' perceptions of good outcomes and their perceptions of the relationship as one in which there exists a mutuality of goals and expectations, a strong bond, and reciprocally held positive feelings.

A 20th-century shift in scientific paradigms—one which recognized that the observer inevitably influences the nature of the phenomenon being observed—also indirectly paved the way for the emergence of relationally oriented therapies. While many of Freud's colleagues, including those who immigrated to the United States, attempted to modify and extend the principles or application of classical analysis, they tended to do so within the context of outdated scientific models. It was Harry Stack Sullivan, founder of the interpersonal school of psychiatry, who developed a participant–observation model that was implicitly based on a 20th-century view of interactional processes. Sullivan's work, and that of many other theorists who followed, acknowledges the contributions of both therapist and patient to the therapeutic process and emphasizes the importance of their reciprocal influence.

Yet another reason for many contemporary therapists' adoption of a more relationally oriented psychotherapy—one in which issues of openness and disclosure (on the part of both participants) are inevitably addressed—may be located in the profession's response to the pressures of managed care. As a reaction against the mechanized, impersonal, short-term prescriptive approach favored by managed care companies, many therapists have vigorously renewed their belief in and commitment to a psychotherapy that is more oriented toward treating the whole person rather than only his or her symptoms. Of course, this is not true of everyone; some therapists have responded to these pressures by adopting more symptom-oriented approaches. Still, there is something about strong pressures to change, or adopt a certain approach to one's work, that can catalyze deep thinking about one's values and what one expects and needs from the practice and process of psychotherapy.

Regardless of the exact reasons for the movement toward a more relationally oriented therapy, one consequence of this trend is greater clinical and research attention paid to the issue of therapist disclosure. Clinically, it appears that adherents of most forms of psychotherapy have adopted practices regarding therapist disclosures that are far less restrictive than traditional norms. Empirically (see next chapter), studies investigating the types, frequencies, and consequences of therapist disclosures have increased dramatically over the past few years.

The history of therapist self-disclosure reflects long-standing divisions in the field. As with most clinical debates, Freud stands squarely at the center of the storm. His rare but persuasive writings on analytic technique contain decrees against which most psychoanalytically oriented therapists have traditionally measured the purity of their clinical practices. Arguably, most contemporary psychodynamically oriented clinicians can be placed into one of three main categories of allegiance: classical analysts who strive to maintain Freudian ideals of nondisclosure; so-called wild analysts whose idiosyncratic disclosure practices have tested the boundaries of therapeutic practice; and those in the middle of this hypothetical continuum whose belief in the healing powers of the therapeutic relationship guides their moderate use of moderately intimate disclosures. Needless to say, this division is rough at best; like most systems that attempt to categorize complex phenomena, this one finesses the real-life fluidity of seemingly discrete theoretical positions. Nevertheless, this proposed trichotomy of positions provides a convenient framework for presenting a chronological account of the topic while paying homage to the controversy it has ignited.

THE CLASSICAL POSITION

> The doctor should be opaque to his patients, and like a mirror, should show them nothing but what is shown to him.
> —FREUD (1912, p. 117)

The classical position, as espoused by Freud and perpetuated by his followers, purports an inverse relationship between analyst and patient self-disclosure: the more the analyst reveals of him or herself, the less the patient will. To justify this perspective, Freud (1912) emphasized two related risks: the contamination of the transference and the intrusion of reality at the expense of fantasy. Therapist disclosure—indeed, any unnecessary intrusion of the therapist's needs, personal beliefs, or experiences—diminishes the patient's ability to reveal fully his or her inner world, especially those irrational or shameful elements. Thus, Freud (1912) cautioned against analysts' bringing "their own individuality" into the therapy because "the resolution of the transference . . . , one of the main tasks of the treatment, is made more difficult by an intimate attitude on the doctor's part, so that any gain there may be at the beginning is more outweighed at the end" (p. 118). Freud acknowledged that certain aspects of the analyst could not be concealed, including gender, approximate age, physical appearance, and health; he was also aware that patients might learn something personal about the analyst from mutual acquaintances, including other patients. These were thought to be regrettable if inevitable aspects of the analytic situation.

In his writings on technique, Freud established a special posture, role, and task for the analyst. These three components, if properly executed, would guard against the dangers of analyst interference in the treatment. The *posture*, then considered novel but now the stuff of stereotypes and popular culture, consists of analytic neutrality, abstinence, and anonymity—in essence, the infamous "blank screen" situated behind the equally infamous couch. The *role* of the analyst was to reflect all that the patient projected onto the carefully cultivated blank screen. Lastly, the primary *task* that Freud charged classical analysts with was interpretation—especially the interpretation of the transference that originated in the patient's childhood and reemerged within the facilitative environment of the analytic relationship.

It is not difficult to see how these prescribed positions determine the classical stance toward therapist self-disclosure. Any statement or behavior that violates neutrality, anonymity, and abstinence, and any intervention that deviates from facilitating patient projections or interpreting the emerging transference, runs the risk of contaminating the treatment. In fact, therapist disclosure reverses the roles of therapist and patient such that the *former's* associations provide the data of the treatment rather than the latter's (Aron, 1996). Furthermore, therapist disclosures may burden patients, shift attention to analysts' needs and feelings, foreclose learning opportunities by inhibiting fantasies, cause vulnerable patients to overly identify with their analysts, and, under certain circumstances, seem seductive (Aron, 1996; Hanly, 1998; Tillman, 1988). For all these reasons, classical analysts have assiduously avoided purposeful disclosures. Many have even refused to acknowledge mistakes, a tack that most contemporary therapists would now regard as inappropriate and as countertherapeutic.

Compared to the devotion with which he developed and amended his metapsychological tenets, Freud's technical writings seem almost insignificant. Yet, unlike his theories of the psyche, which were always subject to revision, Freud's few writings on analytic technique were definitive, unyielding, and, by his own admission, largely couched in the negative (Grubrich-Simitis, 1986). Indeed, he did not revisit or alter these views despite a later admission that the lack of "elasticity" of these pronouncements would "have to be revised someday but without setting aside the obligations" (cited in Grubrich-Simitis, 1986, p. 270).

Although the number of classical analysts has dwindled in recent years, there are still those who pledge allegiance to traditional Freudian ideals. On the more conservative end of the spectrum is Langs (1975), who argues that the maintenance of boundaries is the most critical determinant of therapeutic outcome and that interventions other than strict interpretation hinder the healing process. Although Langs acknowledges that certain analyst disclosures are inevitable (e.g., those that emanate from office decor or dress or linguistic style), he recommends strict abstinence from deliberate self-revelation. Etchegoyen (1991) concurs with Langs' disapproval of deliberate self-disclosure, arguing that the patient, not the analyst, should provide the material and associations for therapy. Similarly, Epstein (1995) warns analysts not to demystify themselves for their patients; this, in effect, does patients' work for them. In this regard, a former student of mine, currently in analysis, reported to me the following interchange in a class she was taking at a prestigious analytic institute. The instructor noted that after professional events at this institute (e.g., case conferences, lectures), it was now fairly common practice for analysands to follow their analysts out to their cars to chat and say a brief goodbye. He further stated that he saw no harm in this practice and that it might even provide useful material for analytic sessions. She alone of all her classmates argued against this position, claiming that it interfered with the primitive, relatively pure, and analytically important fantasies she had of her analyst.

Reflecting a somewhat less conservative position (though fully within orthodox bounds), Lane and Hull (1990) concluded that affective disclosures should be used sparingly, that neutrality is the best therapeutic posture, and that analyst self-disclosure more often than not impedes the progress of the treatment. However, they conceded that certain revelations can be useful, and described their overall attitude toward self-disclosure as one of "tempered restraint" (p. 43).

EVALUATING THE CLASSICAL POSITION ON DISCLOSURE

Although interpreted in too doctrinaire a fashion by too many of his followers—especially in light of the fact that his own behavior contradicted the orthodoxy of his writings—it is useful to keep in mind that Freud made his clinical recommendations with the patients' best interests in mind, seeking to protect them from undue intrusions on their journey toward cure (or at least self-knowledge). He also believed that boundary violations of any sort, however well-intentioned, might jeopardize treatment by causing patients to become "insatiable" in their pursuit of personal favors and intimacies from their therapist (1912, p. 117).

A contemporary argument against self-disclosure is that analysts cannot understand fully their motivations for such behavior and are therefore liable to blur their needs with those of their patients, creating confusion for both parties in the process (e.g., Hanly, 1998; Langs, 1975). That is, despite their highly practiced psychological-mindedness and openness toward self-understanding, analysts are unlikely to comprehend fully their motivations for disclosing, including their desire for narcissistic gratification, wish to save the client from the arduous work of analysis, and need to avoid feelings of boredom in the room. Aron (1996) conveys this point well when he notes that "deliberate self-revelations are always highly ambiguous and are enormously complicated. Our own psychologies are as complicated as our patients' and our unconsciouses no less deep" (p. 88).

In sum, there are three major objections to therapist disclosure: at least at its extremes, it may be harmful to patients and clinicians alike, whereas neutrality and abstinence protect both parties; its effects do not lend themselves to easy prediction; and therapists' motivations for disclosure are nearly impossible to understand and may reflect their own needs as much as those of their patients.

On the other hand, Freud's stance toward therapist disclosure has received a fair amount of criticism from therapists within the classical tradition and extensive criticism from without. Whereas some traditional analysts contend that therapist neutrality and nondisclosure *prevent* harm, critics argue that such a posture actually *causes* harm. For example, some have argued that the blank-screen mentality of the classical analyst is a form of "professional hypocrisy" that promotes aloofness and distance (Ferenczi, 1933, p. 158; Lane & Hull, 1990). The unwitting effect of the classical stance, Ferenczi contended, is a reenactment of the very parent–child traumas that led to the patient's illness. Jacobs (1999) provides a more moderate argument in this regard, stating that therapist abstinence is especially inappropriate when treating patients with secretive and nonresponsive parents; in such cases, the traditional analytic role may inhibit rather than liberate patients. Others (e.g., Aron, 1996) have suggested that neutrality and nondisclosure "tantalize" patients into wanting to learn more about their analysts, resulting in the very shift in focus—from patient to analyst—that the classical stance was meant to prevent.

In addition, some critics have averred that the "blank-screen" posture, with its attendant nondisclosing stance, is essentially defensive. It protects analysts by inhibiting patient criticism (Ferenczi, 1933), promoting excessive idealization (Renik, 1995), and moderating analysts' own libidinal impulses toward patients (Gerson, 1996). Aron (1996) adds that it is far easier for analysts to think of therapy as unidirectional, as the blank-screen position suggests, rather than acknowledge the complex bidirectional ("two-person") nature of the therapeutic relationship.

Finally, many critics have argued that Freud's call for abstinence, neutrality, and anonymity is simply impossible to fulfill. This is especially true of self-disclosure, which most analysts now agree is inevitable (Aron, 1996; Hanly, 1998; Singer, 1997). Even strict technical interpretations are self-revealing, and most patients come to realize this. Perhaps Aron said it best when he remarked, "You can sit, but never hide, behind the couch" (1996, p. 97).

REBELS, REVOLUTIONARIES, AND WILD ANALYSTS: THE RADICAL POSITION

> Certain phases of mutual analysis represent the complete renunciation of all . . . authority on both sides: [Patient and analyst] give the impression of two equally terrified children who compare their experiences, and because of their common fate understand each other completely and instinctively try to comfort each other.
> —FERENCZI (1933, p. 156) [on his new therapeutic technique]

Mutual analysis, unexpurgated disclosures of love and hate, and social relationships with patients: This is the stuff of the so-called wild analysts, revolutionary therapists whose clinical practices stand in stark contrast to Freud's recommendations. Various eyewitness accounts (see Momigliano,

1987) suggest that, contrary to popular belief, such controversial clinical practices did not merely occur on the periphery of mainstream analysis; rather, a culture of subversion coexisted with classical psychoanalysis, and often proponents of one school were members of the other.

For example, as early as 1923, Georg Groddeck (the originator of the term "id") was persuading Ferenczi to accept the benefits of role reversal between therapist and patient in psychoanalysis (Aron, 1996). Carl Jung attempted mutual analysis with a patient 15 years before Ferenczi's infamous clinical experiments; moreover, not only did Jung suggest that his psychic health benefited from these encounters, but Freud himself "heartily approved of the doctor ceding medical authority to a clearly disturbed patient and then accepting the patient's diagnosis of what ailed him" (Bair, 2003, p. 142). Much later, Searles (1975) continued the spirit, although not the literal practice, of mutuality by focusing on the patient's capacity to analyze his or her therapist.

In fact, Freud himself was the first violator of his own precepts. The same man who advocated professional distance was also known to show personal pictures to patients, lend books, give gifts, provide financial assistance, chat and gossip about family and colleagues, discourse on art and archeology, conduct analysis in the presence of his dog, and analyze his friends and daughter (Gay, 1989; Goldstein, 1994; Hill & Knox, 2002; Johnston & Farber, 1996; Lane & Hull, 1990; Momigliano, 1987). According to Momigliano (1987):

> He seems to have had no objection to speaking perfectly freely on any subject proposed to him by the patients; indeed, he responded to all their varied remarks and questions patiently and perhaps with a certain pleasure, on the reality level—and everyone asked him many questions, as if they were eager to profit from their relations with Freud to obtain from him explanations of the theory and technique of psychoanalysis, but also know his personal opinions on political, artistic, and religious matters, his colleagues, friends and enemies and even his personal life. (p. 382)

As a world celebrity whose writings were widely accessible to his patients, Freud realized that anonymity was not an option for him. However, neutrality and abstinence within the boundaries of analytic sessions were options, but apparently not chosen. In Freud's defense, many of these documented boundary violations occurred early in his career, in the formative years of psychoanalysis. In addition, there is something inherently anachronistic and perhaps unfair about applying contemporary ethical and clinical standards to Freud's early professional behavior. Furthermore, Freud did have an awareness of the limits of these personal gestures with patients, refusing, for example, to play cards with Marie Bonaparte because "it's too intimate" (Momigliano, 1987, p. 380).

Still, the forcefulness of Freud's 1912 writings on analyst opacity stands in stark contrast to his self-disclosing behavior, leaving us to wonder which set of values he most truly believed in. The critics such as Crews (1984) have noted, often quite vehemently, that Freud often exhibited a "Do as I say, not as I do" attitude, a stance that giants in many fields have adopted. Thus, notwithstanding his published dicta, Freud holds a secure if ironic place in the pantheon of iconoclastic analysts. As Peter Gay (1989) noted, "Freud played this game with the rest" (p. 235).

Despite deviations from his own rules, Freud was hardly considered radical. However, others, like Ferenczi, were viewed this way and denounced by the analytic establishment as excessive, unethical, and unwise. While there is some truth to these charges, so-called radical or wild analysts were not simply gratuitous rebels, violating boundaries for the thrill of defiance. Many, Ferenczi included, conducted their bold experiments out of genuine concern for the well-being of their patients. Frustrated by the constrictions imposed on analysts in the classical tradition, these clinicians sought to demystify the role of the analyst by placing different aspects of their personalities at the patient's disposal. These innovative and free-spirited clinicians were devoted to the spirit of analytic theory but not to the letter of its techniques, and they openly propounded the benefits of increased therapist disclosure.

In this section, two historically prominent proponents of analyst self-disclosure are discussed: Sandor Ferenczi and Masud Khan.

Sandor Ferenczi

Alternatively branded as excessive and courageous, flawed and heroic, Ferenczi is the original "enfant terrible" of psychoanalysis (Aron, 1996). Indeed, many unorthodox analysts have invoked Ferenczi's clinical experiments as justification for their own incursions into controversial therapeutic territory. And what a rich heritage to invoke! Ferenczi's legacy includes forays into "active" techniques, frequent and explicit countertransference disclosures, and reciprocal analyses of patients (Aron, 1996; Johnston & Farber, 1996). His experiments are especially noteworthy because they occurred within the context of his intense but tenuous friendship with Freud.

Despite his admiration of Freud, and his desperate need for the master's approval, Ferenczi (1926) was explicit regarding his disagreements with classical technique. One major problem with psychoanalysis, he noted, was its marked passivity: "Analysis demands no *activities* from the patient except punctual appearance at the hours of treatment. . . . The patient must comport himself passively during his 'midwifery of thought' " (p. 200). To energize his treatments and to effect a quicker cure, Ferenczi developed what he called the "active technique." This entailed the therapist's purposeful and insistent issuing of "commands and prohibitions" to guide the therapy into a more concrete synthesis of intellectual and affective insights. Examples include encouraging a patient to write poetry, prohibiting free associations in favor of directed discussions, and confronting resistances until affective breakthroughs occur (setting the foundation for much later developments in short-term dynamic psychotherapy). "Activity," Ferenczi concluded, "stimulates the ego," exacerbates symptoms (so that they can be dealt with more readily), and facilitates the expression of previously repressed material.

Another objection that Ferenczi harbored toward psychoanalysis, in addition to its passivity, involved the stance of the analyst. Anonymity and neutrality, in his view, are merely forms of aloofness, and abstinence is tantamount to withholding. In his writings on mutual analysis, he noted that "any kind of secrecy, whether positive or negative . . . makes the patient distrustful; he detects from little gestures . . . the presence of affects, but cannot gauge their . . . importance" (1932, p. 11). Thus, he believed that, in inhibiting their personalities, subjectivities, and countertransference, analysts risked reviving the very traumas and affective failures that brought patients into therapy in the first place (Aron, 1996; Dupont, 1988).

Moreover, according to Ferenczi, the traditional analytic posture initiates a vicious cycle in the therapy: perceiving the therapist's anonymity and abstinence as forms of kindness or acceptance, patients repress their own criticisms of the analyst. In turn, therapists mask their true feeling, both positive and negative, toward their patients, and a culture of denial, separation, and misunderstanding inevitably evolves. To counter this grim scenario, Ferenczi (1932) suggested a new model of analysis in which "the tears of doctor and of patient mingle in a sublimated communion, which perhaps finds its analogy only in the mother–child relationship. And this is the healing agent [that] . . . surrounds the personality . . . with a new aura of vitality and optimism" (p. 65).

Mutual analysis rests on the assumption that, by laying bare their own weaknesses, foibles, and feelings, analysts are able to lift the veil of secrecy in the therapeutic relationship, cultivate greater trust and faith in the dyad, and encourage patients to explore repressed, painful, and previously unassimilated parts of themselves (Aron, 1996; Dupont, 1988). The curative ingredient of the process presumably lies in the analyst's willingness to expose him- or herself to the very vulnerabilities that patients experience in their therapeutic work. In so doing, the analyst attempts to normalize patients' experiences as well as provide a context in which each can relate to the other with "greater assurance" (Dupont, 1988, p. xxi).

Mutual analysis was actually the result of an argument Ferenczi had with one of his patients (Elizabeth Severn) who accused him of having unresolved conflicts that hindered his ability to treat her. Severn perceived Ferenczi as unempathic and indifferent to her pain—an allegation that, given Ferenczi's need for warmth and tenderness, could not have gone unheeded. Thus began a tumultuous experiment into reciprocal therapy, lasting from January 1932 to June 1933, in which Ferenczi and Severn alternated the role of analyst and patient. Each was to openly and candidly reveal to the other his or her innermost conflicts, feelings, and thoughts.

Although he began this enterprise with reservations, Ferenczi was initially pleased with its results. On January 17, 1932, he wrote, "This free discussion with the patient provides a kind of liberation and relief for the analyst in comparison with the activity favored until now" (p. 13). Severn, too, benefited at first from this experiment, which, Ferenczi noted, is less demanding, more genial, and "allows the patient to confess hitherto unconscious affects" (p. 14). At its best, then, mutual analysis facilitated an undoing of painful empathic failures in Ferenczi and Severn's relationship. Each became a "good object" to the other, supplying the tenderness and affection that were so notably absent in their early years. Initially, it seemed as though Ferenczi's eschewing of traditional analytic roles provided a mutually corrective experience that stood in triumphant opposition to Freudian guidelines.

As the experiment progressed, however, its benefits diminished in comparison to the enormous problems that it posed. On March 29, 1932, Ferenczi noted in his diary that Severn grew angry with him because he allowed himself to be analyzed first. "The analysis of the analysand must not be interrupted," he cautioned, and thus imposed the first of a series of limitations on the previously unrestricted endeavor. Several days later, Ferenczi's frustration mounted as he realized that, having spent 2 consecutive days being analyzed himself, "the patient has succeeded in escaping from analysis entirely" (p. 73).

For the next 2 months, the mutual analysis continued its downward spiral. Ferenczi, admitting to feeling humiliated, subordinated, and exhausted by the endeavor, finally announced its end. On June 3, 1932, Ferenczi concluded, with despair: "Mutual analysis: only as a last resort! Proper analysis by a stranger, without any obligation, would be better" (p. 115).

Freud (1912) was concerned with the propensity of "young and eager analysts" to abandon neutrality in favor of intimacy in order to further the healing process. Ferenczi's experiment with mutual disclosure might seem to have corroborated Freud's admonitions. Still, the adverse consequences of establishing a position on the radical edge of the disclosure continuum do little or nothing to refute the wisdom of assuming a position somewhere in the middle of this continuum.

Masud Khan

I have never realized that you were not only mean and cruel, but also lazy!
—KHAN (1986, p. 636) [to an analysand]

In his analysis of "Mr. Roberts," Khan (1986) used self-disclosure in a manner unlike any analyst before him. Whereas Ferenczi used self-revelation systematically and deliberately, treating it as a therapeutic tool within a clinical experiment, Khan dispensed with any such formalities and seemed to disclose simply because he thought it appropriate and clinically useful. He acted as if he should not have to be constrained by anyone else's rules. He invoked a recent bout with cancer ("I had been fighting death for two years") to justify a new stance of "Now I make the demands, not my patients" (p. 637). Some noteworthy examples from the case of Mr. Roberts include:

- Revealing details of his struggles with cancer.
- Disclosing news of his brother's death, which "changed my whole outlook on life, and I knew my patients would sense it" (p. 643).
- Sharing challenging observations, such as "You don't look like one of the upper classes to me" (p. 632).
- Calling his patient's apparent bluff about suicidality: "If that's true, I should have been attending your funeral months ago, and not listening to you telling me this damnable yarn today" (p. 636).

Although the shock value of such statements is undeniable, Khan's intentions in making them were less definitively gratuitous than one might assume. Mr. Roberts, the recipient of these disclosures, was a rigid, highly manipulative passive–aggressive man whose lack of spontaneity originated in his relationship with his oppressive mother. Attempting to break this pattern, Khan countered his patient's provocative behavior with equally provocative statements. Like Ferenczi, Khan adopted a therapeutic style that foreshadowed some aspects of contemporary short-term dynamic psychotherapy.

Khan's rationalization for his behavior, one that echoed Ferenczi's reasons for conducting mutual analysis, involved demystifying the person of the analyst: "Analysts rarely speak about events in their personal life that affect their work mutatively. . . . It is not a question of transference or countertransference, but actually real, lived life that makes our fatedness or destiny, and about which we are often somewhat devious, both with ourselves and others" (p. 644).

Still, one wonders about the extent to which Mr. Roberts' clinical problems suffice as explanations for Khan's work. The overall tone of his article chronicling this work—proud, self-aggrandizing, and defiant ("he could not get the better of me" [p. 648])—combined with his professed affinity for the neglected affect of outrage, suggests more narcissistic motives and thus undermines his contribution to a greater understanding of how and when self-disclosure may be used effectively in clinical work.

EVALUATING THE MERITS
OF THE "RADICAL" POSITION

Arguably, the most enduring benefit of these innovators' efforts has been an increased appreciation of the therapeutic relationship, or, more specifically, the analyst's active presence in the relationship. Radical clinicians, including Ferenczi and Khan, shared a conviction that patient growth and healing accrue as a result of a relationship in which both parties openly acknowledge their thoughts, needs, feelings, and wish for contact with the other. Their experiments with boundary manipulation, mutual analysis, and therapist self-disclosure paved the way for short-term dynamic psychotherapy, humanistic/existential psychotherapies, and the 1960s human potential movement. In turn, many of the tenets of humanistic psychotherapy established the basis for current trends in relational psychoanalysis. Thus, while the excesses of these more radical therapists have been consistently denounced, their extreme positions have served to move the acceptable range of therapist disclosures closer to a point that most therapists find comfortable and helpful. Similarly, radical innovators have likely helped close the discrepancy between what therapists say they disclose and what they actually do disclose.

Criticisms of radical self-disclosure have centered on three points: that it is unfeasible and unrealistic; that it is harmful; and that it serves the analyst's needs rather than the patient's. The argument regarding unfeasibility is that total therapist disclosure is virtually impossible at any given moment and truly impossible in the long run. This line of thinking is somewhat parallel to that proposed in regard to patients: that "full" or "total" disclosure is more an ideal than a reality, and that the full gamut of conscious thoughts and feelings can never be expressed at any given moment. Gestalt therapists endorse a similar concept in contending that the full richness of the here and now can only be experienced and not verbalized. In this regard, too, Aron (1996) wisely points out that "full disclosure is never an option [for therapists]. . . . We are always concealing as we reveal" (p. 132). Just as the classical analyst cannot be entirely anonymous, the radical analyst cannot be fully known in the treatment. Could the degree of openness championed by some analysts ever be maintained? As Ferenczi (1932) ultimately acknowledged, "Mutual analysis is nonsense, also an impossibility" (p. xxii).

The notion of "harmfulness" is that full disclosure potentially compromises the sense of safety of patients, especially the more vulnerable ones. It can feel too intimate, too unclear as to where the intimacy may lead. Some patients experience high degrees of therapist disclosure as sexually provocative, fearing that mutual emotional and intellectual disclosures might lead to physical intimacy. Research on sexual intimacies between patients and therapists provides some justification for this fear: Sexual encounters often begin with therapist disclosures of strong personal feelings about the patient (Epstein, 1994; Simon, 1989). More generally, without the holding environment provided by firm and clear boundaries, more disturbed patients can experience dangerous regressions—the ground just doesn't feel as secure as it needs to be. In addition, therapists may be placed in a vulnerable position as a result of uninhibited disclosures. As noted earlier, Freud (1912) warned that patients might expect, even demand, ever greater personal disclosures from their therapists.

Some also believe that therapist disclosures ultimately serve the therapist's needs and interests rather than the patient's. What motivates any analyst to espouse a technique or theoretical stance? Some have argued that Freud's insistence upon analytic neutrality, anonymity, and abstinence was little more than his way of keeping an overactive libido in check. Similarly, radical analysts have been accused of cultivating clinical postures that serve their unmet needs first and foremost. Ferenczi was raised by cold, withholding parents; his determination to undo parentally inflicted traumas in his patients by sharing with them his own similar experiences renders his motivations questionable (Aron, 1996). And Khan's acerbic countertransferential disclosures seem motivated by his own extraordinary competitiveness: "I was a much cuddled infant/child, who grew up, very precociously, to speak seven languages, be a champion international rider and squash player. So he could not get the better of me" (1986, p. 648). Clearly, it was important that he, not Mr. Roberts, "win" their battle of wills.

More generally, indiscriminate therapist disclosure may reflect the therapist's own narcissism (e.g., need to be heard, seen, experienced as an equal partner in a dialogue). If perceived this way by the patient, therapist disclosures can damage the relationship and actually inhibit rather than facilitate patient disclosure.

A "MIDDLE" POSITION: THE RISE OF THE RELATIONAL/INTERSUBJECTIVE SCHOOL

The theoretical and clinical shift toward the primacy of relationships rather than drives began in Freud's lifetime. Some (e.g., Reisner, 1991) view Freud as the first object relations theorist, contending that this aspect of his theoretical writings has long been underappreciated. Most scholars, however, designate Melanie Klein as the first true object relations thinker, and link the publication of her theories regarding infant relationships with fantasized others to the emergence of an object relational movement that gained rapid momentum over the last half of the 20th century. Although most of the early object relations and interpersonal theorists had little to say directly about therapist self-disclosure, many made critical indirect contributions to the ongoing debate. The contributions of several of these prominent figures—Klein, Winnicott, Fairbairn, and Sullivan—are worth briefly considering in this regard.

Melanie Klein

Although her espousal of analytic neutrality and abstinence aligns her more closely with classical rather than relational ideals, Klein nevertheless influenced current perspectives on analyst self-disclosure. Positioning the object (person), not the drives, as the fundamental psychic entity, Klein refocused clinical interest on the therapeutic object par excellence: the analyst. In the Kleinian model, drives are merely the vehicles for relationships; they steer individuals toward contact with important others.

As the most significant object in a patient's life, the analyst is often the target of a host of primitive defensive strategies that accompany the drive toward relationships. Especially important is the concept of projective identification, the splitting and subsequent deflection of intolerable affects onto another. Thus, in clinical situations, a therapist's affects may or may not have originated within him- or herself; strong emotional experiences may reflect the expression of a patient's infantile defenses. Within the Kleinian model, analysts were no longer seen as possessing a neutral, objective reality; however detached and uninvolved they might appear within the analytic session, their psychic realities were now vulnerable to "hostile takeover" through a patient's defensive maneuvers. Why reveal affective data to a patient when such affects may, in fact, actually be the *patient's* disowned and dissociated feelings (Mitchell, 1995)? Therapist disclosure, then, may foreclose the patient's capacity for recognizing and owning that which he or she has disavowed. Nevertheless, the critical point here is that, in recasting analysts as susceptible to a patient's intrapsychic conflicts and desires, Klein opened the formerly closed clinical system and laid the foundation for later perspectives that emphasized the value of focusing on the mutually influential nature of patient and therapist interactions.

D. W. Winnicott

Arguably the most widely read and most clinically influential of the British object relations theorists, Winnicott was concerned with the analytic environment and held the analyst responsible for creating and preserving the ideal climate for mental growth. Winnicott's developmental theories provided the basis for his clinical style. "There is no such thing as a baby," he asserted (1952, p. 99), but rather only a "nursing couple" whose joint relatedness forms the basis of a nurturing holding environment that serves to anticipate and meet the infant's needs. The therapeutic dyad, for Winnicott, is a re-creation of this original nursing couple. The analyst/mother provides the ideal holding environment, carefully protecting the infant/patient from intrusion and impingement. Analysis aims to supply all of the patient's developmental provisions that were previously unmet in infancy. Thus, the curative aspects in Winnicott's vision of psychoanalysis lie not in the therapist's interpretations but rather in the mutual interplay of the analytic dyad, the analyst's presentation of missing parental provisions, and the minimization of intrusions that threaten to falsify the patient's evolving self.

From his work with schizophrenics and other severely disturbed patients, Winnicott concluded that a certain degree of therapist self-disclosure is appropriate with these populations, primarily because their lack of psychic organization makes a seemingly distant and withholding therapist unbearable (Winnicott, 1965). However, Winnicott was far more conservative when it came to self-disclosure with less disturbed patients. This stemmed from his emphasis on the importance of cultivating an environment free from unnecessary intrusion (Jackson, 1990). Although he is often quoted for a remark he made to one of his patients ("I really hate your mother"; Little, 1985), Winnicott was not especially self-revealing in his clinical work. He did, however, reinterpret the analytic role to allow for the types of influence (e.g., more open expressions of caring and empathy) that subsequent generations of relational therapists have achieved more directly through self-disclosure.

W. R. D. Fairbairn

Unlike Klein and Winnicott, who maintained varying degrees of allegiance to Freud and the drive/structure paradigm (Greenberg & Mitchell, 1983), Fairbairn (1946) made no bones about his disagreements with the classical tradition. "[The] libido," he wrote, "is not primarily pleasure-seeking, but object-seeking" (p. 30). He thus emphasized the analyst's need to establish rapport. As Guntrip (1975) recalled hearing from Fairbairn in his analysis with him, "You can go on analyzing forever and get nowhere. It's the personal relation that's therapeutic" (p. 145).

Fairbairn's vision suggests that the decision to disclose must occur on an individual basis. If the patient is highly identified with the rejecting mother, for example, then withholding a disclosure may perpetuate early trauma. On the other hand, for patients who pathologically seek gratification, analyst self-disclosures may cause more harm than good. Although his exact beliefs about analyst self-revelation were unarticulated, Fairbairn's explicit renunciation of the drive/structure model, his criticism of the abstinent and neutral blank-screen analyst, and his emphasis on objects rather than pleasure-seeking drives added to the foundation for future relational perspectives on therapist self-disclosure.

Harry Stack Sullivan

While the British object relations theorists were steering psychoanalysis away from the Freudian drive/structure model, American psychiatrist Harry Stack Sullivan was initiating his own break from the classical tradition. As noted earlier, his emphasis on participation–observation was instrumental in establishing a new model for understanding the therapeutic process. Objecting to Freud's focus on intrapsychic forces, Sullivan attempted to broaden psychoanalysis by focusing on the contextual determinants of personality. The interpersonal approach that Sullivan championed was based on the assumption that personality emerges as a function of the quality and nature of one's interpersonal interactions; relatedly, then, the most important determinant of therapeutic outcome is the personal relationship between analyst and patient (Aron, 1996; Greenberg & Mitchell, 1983).

Opposed to detachment and neutrality, Sullivan (1953) envisioned the analyst as a coparticipant in the therapeutic process. He believed that such participation necessarily included self-revelation. Along with such notable contemporaries as Frieda Fromm-Reichmann and Clara Thompson, Sullivan emphasized the value of overt frankness about the analyst's role in the analytic process, including the need at times to acknowledge mistakes, feeling states (e.g., irritability), and oversights due to personal problems (Papouchis, 1990; Thompson, 1956). Sullivan's work inspired his followers to advocate strongly for mutuality in psychoanalysis (Aron, 1996) and to reveal relevant countertransferential reactions as they occur throughout the treatment (Mitchell & Black, 1995).

As influential as Winnicott, Fairbairn, and Sullivan were, the change from a one- to a two-person psychology became fully realized in the intersubjective and relational movements of psychoanalysis. Within these closely related paradigms, new perspectives on the role of the analyst, the value of countertransference, and therapist self-disclosure were consolidated and brought to the foreground of contemporary psychoanalytic therapy.

CONTEMPORARY RELATIONAL ANALYSIS AND THE INTERSUBJECTIVE MOVEMENT

Within any psychoanalytic situation . . . two subjective worlds are continually self-revealing and attempting to hide
—ORANGE AND STOLOROW (1998, p. 532)

Like their imaginative predecessors, contemporary relationally oriented psychoanalytic therapists advocate for a reexamination of traditional analytic ideals regarding boundary maintenance and therapist influence. However, unlike the so-called wild analysts—those who willfully broached analytic dicta in order to push the boundaries and scope of practice—this group's approach to therapist participation in the treatment has generally evolved slowly and systematically. In fact, it was not until Greenberg and Mitchell's (1983) comprehensive synthesis of several post-Freudian schools of analysis that a more or less unified tradition emerged. Within the theoretical holding environment of "relational analysis," the previously disparate approaches of British object relations theorists, American interpersonalists, and self-psychologists found common ground in their denunciation of drive theory, emphasis on self–other interactions (personal relationships), and the belief in a two-person psychology in which the words and behavior of both participants are examined to determine how they were co-created (Aron, 1996; Greenberg & Cheselka, 1995; Greenberg & Mitchell, 1983).

The therapist's subjectivity and participation in the treatment gained validity in these newer models of analysis; thus, his or her judicious use of self-disclosure became permissible, indeed, often desirable (Fosha, 2000; Gerson, 1996; Goldstein, 1994, 1997; Zeddies, 2000). That is, as the therapeutic system opened and attachments and interpersonal relationships became the focus of clinical inquiry, the analyst's role changed accordingly (Aron, 1996). Analysts could now actively participate in the treatment by using their own subjectivity as both data and as an instrument within the treatment process. Therapist self-disclosure, previously considered an intrusive, contaminating force, now was seen as an intervention that might well enhance the therapeutic relationship and further the search for meaning, truth, and subjective reality (Jackson, 1990). In fact, with but minor exceptions (e.g., Renik, 1995, 1999, 2002), the theorists and schools of thought that comprise this third approach to analyst self-disclosure—the relational/intersubjective perspective—do not embody extreme views regarding self-disclosure. Rather, they exist on a continuum, ranging from permissive tolerance of self-disclosure to explicit endorsement of all or at least some of its elements.

Relational and intersubjective theorists tend to be critical of Freud's vision of the analyst. For example, Orange and Stolorow (1998) challenged Freud's notion that nondisclosure constitutes abstinence and neutrality, arguing that neither the decision to disclose nor withhold is inherently neutral: "Even withholding is a form of communication" (p. 532). In fact, within this new perspective, there are no hard-and-fast rules, no de facto right or wrong positions regarding therapist disclosure; decisions regarding this and all other interventions need to be made on a case-by-case basis (Greenberg & Cheselka, 1995; Orange & Stolorow, 1998). "Self-disclosure," noted Bromberg (1994), "derives its meaning from the ongoing context of the relationship in which it takes place, not from its utility as a 'technique.' . . . If the analyst's choice is motivated by his need to be seen in a certain way (such as honest, accommodating, unsadistic, or innovatively 'free' as an analyst) then self-disclosure becomes a technique" (p. 539). Bromberg's admonition here is reminiscent of a *New Yorker* cartoon wherein one character comments to another about a mutual acquaintance, "He's becoming insufferably 'more transparent than thou.' "

Self-revelation can be both healing and harmful; the quality of the therapeutic relationship and the developmental needs of the patient determine if and when an analyst should engage in self-disclosure. Most importantly, though, the intersubjective–relational perspective has underscored the point that under the right conditions therapist self-disclosure carries with it numerous benefits: resolving treatment impasses (Gerson, 1996; Safran & Muran, 2000), furthering the mutual generation of data (Aron, 1996), assisting clients in formulating previously inchoate and unconscious experiences, and challenging therapists and clients alike to consider what ingredients make the analytic relationship healing (Zeddies, 2000).

SELF-DISCLOSURE IN OTHER PSYCHODYNAMIC MODELS: SELF PSYCHOLOGY, SHORT-TERM DYNAMIC PSYCHOTHERAPIES, AND THE WORK OF OWEN RENIK

Contemporary analytic perspectives on therapist disclosure have been influenced not only by the intersubjective/relational schools, but by self psychology, by various short-term dynamic models, and by the controversial writings of Owen Renik.

Self Psychology

Although contemporary self psychologists (e.g., Goldstein, 1994, 1997) tend to view analyst self-disclosure favorably, Kohut's (1977) stance on this issue is surprisingly consistent with that of Freud. Kohut viewed therapist disclosures as problematic countertransferential intrusions that prematurely expose patients to the analyst's separateness and individuality. That is, by disclosing and thereby becoming more distinct and separate, therapists inhibit patients' salutary perceptions of a self-affirming oneness. For narcissists in particular, Kohut's preferred patient population, premature differentiation from others is destructive and traumatic. Self-disclosure in the Kohutian sense, then, is contraindicated, not because it violates principles of neutrality and abstinence (as in the classical Freudian paradigm), but because it reinforces the separateness of the analyst and patient (Jackson, 1990). Kohut seemed to encourage therapist disclosures only in the admission of technical errors and blatant professional failures.

Contemporary self psychologists, however, have reinterpreted Kohut's formulations. Therapist self-disclosure has been recast as a useful form of empathic resonance (Josephs, 1990). Thus, self psychologists are increasingly suggesting that the content of the therapist's disclosure is less important than his or her actual willingness to engage in the process of disclosure, especially in the case of patients whose narcissism was shaped by detached and withholding parents (Goldstein, 1997). Additionally, a therapist who self-reveals encourages a patient to follow suit. In this sense, Goldstein echoes Jourard's (1971b) earlier ideas regarding the reciprocal effects of self-disclosure. The key to proper use of self-disclosure, according to Goldstein (1994), is correct attunement—finding the tone, words, and body language that reflect the patient's needs. Moreover, refraining from disclosure may result in patients' feeling alienated, rejected, and exposed to the same traumatic early relational patterns that originally gave rise to their narcissism. There is a marked similarity in these ideas to those of Fairbairn.

Short-Term Dynamic Psychotherapies

A host of short-term dynamic therapies (STDPs), largely growing out of the work of Habib Davanloo, have increasingly incorporated the therapist's personality, subjectivity, and affective experiences into the treatment, often in highly structured and carefully orchestrated ways. The theoretical underpinnings of all STDPs originated in Ferenczi's (1926) "active technique," in which he attempted to link cognitively based insights with a simultaneous revival of affect. Liberal use of transference interpretations and countertransference disclosures are hallmarks of the STDP model. McCullough's (1997) short-term anxiety regulating therapy and Fosha's (2000) accelerated experiential dynamic psychotherapy are treatments that, to varying degrees, actively promote therapist self-disclosure.

Short-term anxiety regulating therapy is a model of psychotherapy that attempts to rapidly restructure a patient's defenses, affects, and self–other relationships. To accomplish these goals, the therapist becomes both instrument and catalyst of change. Affective self-disclosures are used, for example, to appeal to patients to relinquish problematic and destructive defenses (McCullough, 1997):

> T: It's really upsetting to see you suffer week after week. How can you
>   bear to continue behaving in ways that bring you so much pain? (p.
>   155)

McCullough (1997) views such disclosures as useful and appropriate for several reasons: They prevent the often more damaging alternative of detachment and withholding; they facilitate the treatment process by providing patients with necessary feedback and information that might otherwise be inaccessible to them; and they keep countertransferential feelings conscious, where they can be examined and monitored. It is an unfortunate consequence of the classical tradition's eschewal of therapist disclosure that such affective expression is still suppressed by some therapists, all the while exerting its influence on patients in subtle but powerful ways.

Fosha (2000) developed accelerated experiential dynamic psychotherapy (AEDP) out of her conviction that affective experiences occurring in the safety of a close relationship inspire change and promote healing. Her treatment model simultaneously builds upon McCullough's use of therapist self-disclosure while elaborating and formalizing its use in a highly prescriptive form. Fosha has identified three types of self-revelations in her work:

1. Affective disclosures, in which the therapist discusses his or her emotional response to the patient, thus acknowledging the patient's impact on the treatment relationship. Examples include disclosing affectionate feelings for patients, or revealing struggles and difficulties in cultivating closeness with them. Fosha believes that these affective disclosures engender awareness of feelings of previously unmet needs for intimacy and closeness with others.

2. Acknowledgment of errors, limitations, and vulnerability. This type of disclosure is useful in establishing a therapist's willingness to engage in the treatment process, and simultaneously liberates the therapist from the shame that often accompanies professional lapses and technical mistakes. It is considered appropriate by practitioners in many contemporary forms of psychodynamic work (Basescu, 1990) and, moreover, has been shown empirically to benefit the relationship (Safran, Muran, Samstag, & Stevens, 2002).

3. Self-disclosures that counteract therapeutic omnipotence (especially appropriate for patients who simultaneously idealize others and devalue themselves). Fosha (2000) argues that such revelations promote healthy differentiation and individuation while empowering patients to recognize their own ego strengths. She provides the following example of this type of disclosure:

> T: I'm so touched [voice trembling with tears]. I have such a sense of love from you. There is something about how we know each other. . . . it is so deep. . . . I'm learning something about the place I go to when I get that look, I'm learning something about it from you [with some tears]. So I want to thank you. (p. 241)

What the STDP model offers to the ongoing self-disclosure debate is a theoretically grounded systematic methodology for meaningfully and logically incorporating the person of the therapist, including his or her affective experiences, into the course of treatment without compromising its psycho-dynamic underpinnings.

Owen Renik

If there is one analyst in the contemporary psychotherapeutic scene who is perceived as an outlier, as a true maverick in regard to self-disclosure, it is Owen Renik. The essential contrariness of Renik's views is made even more apparent by his forceful rhetoric: "We need to begin by not just discarding the principle of analytic anonymity, but by *contradicting* it" (1995, p. 482, emphasis in original).

Like many contemporary analysts, Renik finds fault with the classical position and what he terms the "cloak of anonymity" behind which thera-pists hide (p. 476). Striving for anonymity, Renik (1995) argues, is both defensive and impossible, a fiction disguised as a prohibition against having a personality. Anonymity, from the classical standpoint, prevents patients from paying undue attention to analysts. Yet, Renik (1999) makes the opposite contention: The more that analysts are willing to acknowledge and explore their presence in the therapy, the *less* room they actually con-sume and the *more* room they leave for the patient. His idea here is that awareness of who the therapist is and what he or she is thinking obviates patients' need to fantasize about these subjects and thus leaves greater room for them to focus on their own issues.

Renik is quite clear about his use of self-disclosure, avowing that he is consistently willing to make his own views "explicitly available to the patient" (1999, p. 522). He argues that all analytic interventions require some degree of self-disclosure and that the ultimate effect of judicious self-revelation is that patients will follow suit. Although he recommends that analysts create guidelines about the types of disclosures that promote positive outcome, he is not concerned that the act of self-revelation will lead to exploitation, believing that the analyst's superego will keep his or her impulses in check (Wasserman, 1999).

Putting his theoretical views into practice, Renik advocates an "epi-stemological symmetry" in the analytic situation. In this collaborative ar-rangement, therapist and patient share equal responsibility for full disclosure about the nature of the treatment relationship. In this regard, his ideas (like Fosha's) are quite consistent with Safran and Muran's (2000) model for re-pairing ruptures in the therapeutic alliance, advocating strongly for continu-ous and open processing of the work and the vicissitudes of the relationship.

THE CBT PERSPECTIVE

Before closing this chapter, it seems prudent to consider how proponents of cognitive-behavioral therapy view the role of therapist disclosure. After all, the long-held hegemony of psychodynamic models has been essentially usurped during the past few decades by a similar academic and market-place dominance by CBT perspectives. However, before summarizing the surprisingly scant literature on the use of disclosure by CBT therapists, I'll note a curious but somewhat relevant historical fact. O. Hobart Mowrer, a prominent learning theorist during the middle of the 20th century whose work paved the way for the emergence of behavior therapy (e.g., he invented the buzzer and pad apparatus for the treatment of enuresis) also wrote extensively about religion and the connection between psycho-pathology and personal sin. As a therapist himself, he found that the most effective way to teach personal openness to his clients was by modeling it himself—in his case, by revealing his own past sins.

Albert Ellis views rational-emotive therapy (RET) as both the precur-sor to other forms of CBT and the leading exemplar of the CBT movement. RET holds that, despite differences in character traits, behaviors, thoughts, and feelings, all people struggle with common human problems and all struggle to control emotional responses. In RET, the therapist's role is seen as openly educational. The therapist is encouraged to share his or her own relevant experiences in the realm of emotional control; that is, therapists can and should describe the process of successfully applying RET methods to deal with emotional problems by drawing from personal experience (Dryden, 1990). Therapist disclosures of this kind thus serve a dual pur-pose in RET: They build trust and strengthen the therapeutic alliance by emphasizing the therapist's and client's shared humanity; and they provide an opportunity for modeling the process of solving emotional problems, providing hope for the patient and demonstrating that his or her problems are not insurmountable. Dryden calls this "a coping model of self-disclo-sure" (p. 66)—one that provides clients with practical ways to cope with (rather than unrealistically "master") emotional disturbances.

Aaron Beck, whose own brand of CBT ("cognitive therapy") has much in common with Ellis' RET, also views therapist self-disclosure within educational terms: "Much of the [cognitive] therapist's role consists of drawing on his or her own life experiences and wisdom to propose possi-ble solutions to problems, as well as to educate the patient regarding the nature of intimate relationships" (Beck, Freedman, & Associates, 1990, p. 66). The therapist, says Beck et al., should serve as a role model, providing examples of concrete behaviors and patterns to emulate.

A second type of therapist self-disclosure in CBT involves the therapist's revealing personal reactions to the client. This, too, serves an educational purpose. By providing the client with open and honest feedback about the kinds of responses his or her behavior elicits in the therapist, the therapist is enlightening the client about the ways in which other people may respond to the same behaviors. Beck et al. (1990) suggest that this is an especially appro-priate strategy in dealing with personality-disordered patients. Narcissistic patients, for example, may be consistently blind to the way that others view them. This is, of course, very similar to a psychodynamically oriented therapist's use of countertransferential feelings. However, from a broad-based CBT perspective, disclosing the therapist's immediate personal reactions to the client is viewed as theoretically consistent with the concept of reinforcement (Goldfried, Burckell, & Eubanks-Carter, 2003). Appropriate interpersonal styles can be "rewarded" or positively reinforced by the therapist through disclosure of positive responses to the client, while inappropriate or ineffective ones can be discouraged through (tactful) disclosures of negative therapist responses.

While potentially rife with opportunities for growth, these types of self-disclosures (especially disclosures of negative emotional reactions to the client) must be made with much caution and tact. This is true, of course, of every therapeutic orientation and modality. CBT theorists (e.g., Goldfried et al., 2003) emphasize that such disclosures should be accompanied by statements emphasizing that a person's behavior does not define him or her. For example, a therapist's critical response to a particular behavior should be followed by a statement noting explicitly that this does not imply a dislike of the client as a person. Moreover, disclosures that reflect negative responses to client behaviors should be followed by an assertion of the therapist's conviction that the client is capable of changing these behaviors through the proper and consistent application of cognitive-behavioral methods.

In addition to providing examples of appropriate real-life behavior and offering useful feedback to patients, therapist self-disclosure has been touted by some CBT practitioners (e.g., Walen, DiGiuseppe, & Dryden, 1992) as a means to encourage disclosure in clients. This, of course, has been seen as one of the prime benefits of disclosure in virtually every therapeutic system. Therapist disclosure is seen by CBT clinicians as especially useful in cases where clients have little experience with or skill at disclosure.

The suggested guidelines for using therapist disclosure in CBT differ little from those a psychodynamically oriented therapist might adopt: Keep self-disclosures relevant, elicit feedback from clients about this behavior, and avoid too much self-disclosure. Walen et al. (1992) suggest directly asking patients, "Is there anything about my story that is meaningful for you? How could you apply that?" (p. 64). They also emphasize the potential dangers of overuse of self-disclosure. The tale of the client who exclaims "I'm not paying you good money to hear about your problems" (p. 64) is invoked to urge therapists to exercise restraint and use self-disclosure sparingly in order to maintain its effectiveness. The litmus test for therapist self-disclosure in CBT, as it is in psychodynamically oriented and other therapies, is the answer to the question "Who will benefit from this story?" (Walen et al., 1992, p. 64).

CHAPTER 7

Research Perspectives on Therapist Disclosure

"You confide in me," Breen said. "It seems only fitting that I confide in you."
—BLOCK (1991, cited in Kates, 1997, p. 143)

Knowledge of the soul would unfailingly make us melancholy if the pleasures of expression did not keep us alert and of good cheer.
—MANN (1936, p. 99)

What do therapists tell patients about themselves? How often do they do this? On what bases do they justify disclosures? How do patients view this behavior? And what are the consequences of these disclosures? These are crucial questions to consider, especially because this class of behavior seems to be becoming far more normative among therapists of multiple theoretical persuasions. Yet, as noted in Chapter 6, discussions about therapist disclosure are complicated by the lack of a consensus definition of the term. Similarly, synthesizing the research on the prevalence, nature, and consequences of therapist disclosure is confounded by the diverse range of opinions about how this phenomenon can be understood, measured, and categorized. Despite these controversies, therapist self-disclosure has firmly taken its place in the psychotherapy research community as a variable that is linked to outcome and, as such, merits further empirical study and serious clinical consideration. It should be noted that much of the material in this chapter is based on Hill and Knox's (2002) outstanding review of the research in this area.

In its broadest sense, "self-disclosure" can refer to any behavior, verbal or nonverbal, that reveals information about a person. However, research on therapist self-disclosure has for the most part focused on intentional verbal self-disclosure—the words therapists use to consciously and purposefully communicate private information about themselves to their patients (Simon, 1988). This focus naturally excludes the impact of "unintentional" or nonverbal disclosures (e.g., the therapist's style of dress, facial expressions, or the way his or her office is decorated), an area of increasing interest to many, especially those within the psychodynamic community.

Cozby's (1973) early review of the extant research in this area led him to identify three basic dimensions of therapist self-disclosing behavior: amount, duration, and intimacy level. Although this synthesis proved useful to later researchers, Cozby's definition of disclosure—"any information about himself which Person A communicates verbally to a Person B"—was, in retrospect, too broad. Later, Weiner (1983) described therapist self-disclosure as occurring when therapists offer more than just professional expertise, or when they are purposefully open and genuine with their clients. In Weiner's view, the content of such discourse can include the therapist's feelings, attitudes, opinions, associations, fantasies, experiences, or history. Mathews (1988) offered a similar definition of self-disclosure, one that involves revealing factual information and/or feelings that the therapist has experienced in his or her life, as well as revealing feelings he or she experiences toward the client.

These definitions have been subject to several attempts at refinement. A number of authors (McCarthy & Betz, 1978; Robitschek & McCarthy, 1991; Watkins & Schneider, 1989) have differentiated self-disclosures (statements of factual information about oneself such as personal characteristics) from self-involving responses (statements of emotional reactions to clients that occur within the treatment setting). Self-involving responses have also been termed "immediacy" statements (Knox & Hill, 2003).

Others (e.g., Bridges, 2001) have distinguished between "factual" self-disclosures and countertransference disclosures. This, however, is essentially an example of new wine in old bottles inasmuch as the psychodynamic notion of countertransference disclosures and researchers' notions of "self-involving" or "immediacy" disclosures are virtually indistinguishable. The equivalence is made clear in Wilkenson and Gabbard's (1993) definition of countertransference disclosure as "a form of clinical honesty that focuses on the therapist's experience of the patient in the here-and-now of the session" (p. 282). Regardless of terminology, these kinds of self-disclosures are quite difficult to isolate for research purposes because they tend to blend with the constant give-and-take of typical therapeutic interactions (Busch, 1998; Hanly, 1998; Orange & Stolorow, 1998; Marcus, 1998; Miletic, 1998; Renik, 1999).

Another attempt at definition was provided by Nilsson, Strassberg, and Bannon (1979), who divided disclosures into the "intrapersonal—wherein the therapist reveals information about his or her personal life outside of therapy—and the "interpersonal," in which the therapist reveals feelings about the client's problems or the therapeutic relationship. Clearly, the interpersonal dimension here is similar both to McCarthy and Betz's (1978) self-involving statements and Wilkinson and Gabbard's (1993) countertransference disclosure, whereas the intrapersonal dimension resembles many authors' definition of factual or personal self-disclosure. A variation on the intrapersonal/factual dimension was suggested by Cherbosque (1987), who classified therapist self-disclosure in terms of intrapersonal past (revealing information about past history) and intrapersonal present (information about present personal experiences).

Some authors (e.g., Hoffman & Spencer, 1977) have also differentiated between positive disclosures (sharing favorable information about one's experiences) and negative disclosures (sharing unfavorable information about one's experiences). Still others (e.g., Murphy & Strong, 1972; Watkins & Schneider, 1989) have found it useful to distinguish between "similar statements" (sharing experiences congruent with those of the client) and dissimilar statements (those that are contrary to the client's stated experience). Hill, Mahalik, and Thompson (1989), using slightly different terminology, define similar statements as reassuring and dissimilar statements as challenging. Barrett and Berman (2001) have also noted that self-disclosures can be categorized by whether or not the disclosure is reciprocal—that is, made in response to a similar client disclosure.

Hill and O'Brien (1999) recommended that disclosures be divided into four subtypes: (1) disclosure of facts; (2) disclosure of feelings; (3) disclosure of personal insights; and (4) disclosure of personal strategies. This first subtype—disclosure of facts—clearly corresponds to the definitions of factual self-disclosure presented previously. The other three subtypes can be seen as differentiated aspects of self-involving or countertransferential disclosures. More recently, Knox and Hill (2003) suggested an additional three subtypes, all of which can also be seen as aspects of this latter broad-based self-involving category: disclosures of reassurance/support (e.g., "I too have felt that way"); disclosures of challenge (e.g., "I too have had to struggle with that challenge"); and disclosures of immediacy (e.g., "I'm feeling far away from you now, and wondering if you felt that way in dealing with your family").

Despite the dizzying array of definitions, purposeful therapist self-disclosure can be construed as consisting primarily of two forms:

1. *Factual self-disclosure*: facts or information about the therapist that can be further divided by the length of time spent discussing it, the personal nature of the information, and the amount of information shared. This type of therapist self-disclosure can also be further refined by chronology (whether the information is in the therapist's past or present), whether it is negative or positive, and finally whether it is similar to or different from the patient's experience.

2. *Self-involving (also known as "immediacy" or countertransference disclosures)*: the therapist's articulation of his or her immediate or past feelings or experiences in response to a patient's feelings or experiences. These disclosures may also be further divided into responses directly related to the patient's statements, expressions of the therapist's emotional responses or reactions to the patient in general, and expressions of the therapist's reaction to the patient that are expressly different from the patient's experience. Unfortunately, much of the research in the self-disclosure arena has been unclear regarding which type of disclosure is being studied.

FREQUENCY AND TYPES
OF THERAPIST DISCLOSURE

Several studies have assessed the overall frequency and most common types of therapist self-disclosures. Because there are so many ways of measuring the frequency of disclosures (e.g., therapist surveys, patient reports, assessments made from clinical transcripts) and because the definition of therapist disclosure is so variable, deriving even a "ballpark" figure for the frequency of this behavior has proven elusive. Based on a survey of the research, one might venture to say that it occurs with "moderate" frequency. However, not only is this judgment lacking an operational definition, but also it overlooks the evidence of Hill and colleagues, who argue persuasively that it is a rather uncommon occurrence. One can more confidently state that most therapists occasionally self-disclose but that other behaviors/interventions are far more common in any given session with any given client.

In Berg-Cross' (1984) survey of therapists, self-disclosure appeared to be used at low to moderate levels of frequency with individual item means ranging from 1.49 to 2.98 (where 1 = rarely or never shared with clients, 3 = shared with half of one's clients, and 5 = always shared with clients). Two other studies (Anderson & Mandell, 1989; Edwards & Murdock, 1994) also reported moderate levels of therapist self-disclosure with mean scores of approximately 3 on 5-point scales.

Surveys of psychologists and marriage and family therapists indicate that over 70% use self-disclosure at least occasionally (Brock, 1987; Pope, Tabachnick, & Keith-Spiegel, 1987). Similarly, in Mathews' (1988) study, over 62% of therapists surveyed reported self-disclosing at least occasionally (with 3.6% acknowledging disclosing very often); on the other hand, 25.5% indicated that they never or almost never disclose. Again, the lack of a common metric for phrases like "occasionally" or "almost never" limits the usefulness of these data. Mathews did find that when disclosures occurred 46.1% consisted of feelings that therapists had experienced in their own life, 35% reflected factual information about their own life, and 18.9% were feelings currently experienced toward patients.

In their comprehensive review of the literature, Hill and Knox (2002) found that, across several studies where judges coded transcribed therapy sessions, 1–13% of all therapist interventions (an average of 3.5% per session) were self-disclosures. In one study (Hill et al., 1988), self-disclosures accounted for only 1% of therapists' total responses to clients. However, this behavior received the highest client helpfulness ratings and led to the highest level of emotional experiencing in comparison to eight other therapist response modes, including approval, information, direct guidance, and reflection. Hill et al. hypothesized that therapists' infrequent use of disclosures make these interventions seem especially valuable. These researchers also suggested that disclosures render therapists more "human" to clients and make clients feel less interpersonally vulnerable. This is one of those too rare but wonderful examples of correspondence between researchers' findings and clinicians' beliefs.

Interestingly, the therapists in this study, who were primarily psychodynamically oriented, were more ambivalent than their clients regarding the perceived helpfulness of their self-disclosure—three therapists rated it as the most helpful response mode, whereas the other five therapists in this study rated it as one of the least helpful. Overall, therapists' ratings of the helpfulness of self-disclosure were lower than those of clients.

Frequency of therapist disclosure has also been assessed from the client's perspective. Ramsdell and Ramsdell's (1993) survey found that 58% of former clients reported that their therapist had self-disclosed at least once, and 6% indicated that their therapist had disclosed at least 10 times during the course of therapy. Nevertheless, only 15% indicated that their therapists shared personal information more than two to three times over the course of treatment. In sum, it appears that most therapists—probably in the 65–75% range—occasionally self-disclose personal (factual) information to their patients, although the absolute frequency of this behavior is relatively low. Unfortunately, it has proven difficult to determine the comparative proportion of therapists utilizing self-involving (countertransferential) disclosures. As noted earlier, they tend to be embedded within the fabric of therapeutic dialogue. It is likely, though, that in comparison to personal disclosures self-involving disclosures are used more frequently and by a higher proportion of therapists.

Several studies have found that the frequency of therapist self-disclosure is affected by theoretical orientation. Humanistic/experiential therapists, for example, seem to disclose more than psychoanalytic therapists (Beutler & Mitchell, 1981; Edwards & Murdock, 1994; Simon, 1990). And therapists espousing a feminist orientation are more likely than psychodynamically oriented therapists to disclose their background (including class and religious background, political beliefs, and sexual orientation), endorse the use of self-disclosure, and disclose in order to achieve an egalitarian relationship (Simi & Mahalik, 1997).

Other variables have also been studied in terms of their effects on therapist disclosure. For example, therapists who themselves had a disclosing therapist are especially likely to self-disclose with their own clients (Simon, 1990). On the other hand, the frequency of therapist disclosure is neither affected by gender (Edwards & Murdock, 1994; Robitschek & McCarthy, 1991; Simone, McCarthy, & Skay, 1998), racial/ethnic origins (Edwards & Murdock, 1994), nor years of clinical experience (Simon).

Several studies have examined the content of therapist disclosures. Lane, Farber, and Geller (2001) found that the most frequently disclosed topics included therapists' theoretical orientation, beliefs about the efficacy of therapy, and apologies for clinical mistakes. Some of the least frequently disclosed items in this study included the therapist's dreams, physical attraction to the patient, and personal problems. These findings are generally consistent with previous studies that have indicated that the most frequent disclosures are those that relate to professional background (e.g., training and orientation) while the least common ones focus on therapists' dreams, personal fantasies, and sexual practices and beliefs (Berg-Cross, 1984; Edwards & Murdock, 1994; Robitschek & McCarthy, 1991). Perhaps the most surprising finding in the empirical literature is that reported in Borys and Pope's (1989) oft-quoted survey: 40% of the therapists in their study had disclosed details of current personal stress to a patient. Although Watkins's (1990) review of the literature concluded that therapist disclosures of experiences similar to those of the patient are especially helpful, the practice of revealing aspects of one's personal difficulties seems to run the risk of burdening the patient with the therapist's problems.

Lane et al. (2001) suggested that the most common therapist disclosures are those that give hope to the patient (e.g., beliefs about the efficacy of psychotherapy) and those that strengthen the relationship and repair ruptures in the alliance (e.g., apologies for mistakes). These disclosures would be considered self-involving rather than self-disclosing per se. Their study also asked therapists to rate the extent to which they saw specific disclosures as furthering treatment aims. Disclosures perceived as most advancing treatment included therapists' feelings of respect or admiration for patients, attitudes toward child-rearing, emotional reactions to patients, opinions regarding patients' prognoses, reactions to patients' expressive style, feelings that are similar to those of patients, apologies for mistakes, and strategies for coping with stress. Thus, disclosures perceived as most advancing treatment aims can be seen as providing the patient accurate feedback, positive regard, an enhanced sense of the universality of his or her concerns, or opportunities for modeling appropriate behavior.

Many therapist disclosures (e.g., feelings of admiration and respect for the patient) were rated high by therapists in terms of both frequency and helpfulness in furthering treatment aims. However, in some cases, disclosures with low perceived frequencies were considered effective in advancing treatment aims. For example, whereas a therapist's disclosure of a problem similar to the patient's was rated low to moderate in frequency (contrary to the finding of Borys & Pope, 1989), this disclosure was considered moderately to very helpful. As Hill et al. (1988) and Watkins (1990) have suggested, disclosing certain information too frequently may decrease its potency. One possibility is that frequent disclosures create the perception in patients that the therapist's issues are too often or too reflexively featured in the therapeutic dialogue. Regardless of the exact reason—and more research is needed in this area—it does appear that, at least for certain disclosures (e.g., a therapist's own problems or stress), less may well be more.

Clearly, a therapist's choice of whether, what, and when to disclose is highly individualized and dependent upon a number of different factors, including the therapist's style or theoretical orientation as well as patient diagnosis, length of time in treatment, the nature of the therapeutic relationship, and, most importantly, the exact nature of what is going on in the room at any particular moment. In different clinical situations with different patients, different types of disclosure may be most appropriate. For example, Geller (2001) studied the differences in therapist disclosure when patients were therapists themselves. He found that, while therapists were no more likely than usual to reveal personal/biographical information or personal feelings to patients who are themselves therapists, they did have a greater tendency to discuss current professional issues and research in the field with this type of patient.

REASONS FOR THERAPISTS' DISCLOSURES

Why do therapists disclose? Lane et al. (2001) found that the three most common reasons given by therapists for their use of self-disclosure were strengthening the therapeutic alliance, normalizing the patient's experience, and providing the patient with alternative ways of thinking—findings that are in accord with other literature in the area (e.g., Anderson & Mandell, 1989; Chelune, 1979; Knox, Hess, Peterson, & Hill, 1997; Simon, 1988). Therapists disclose to strengthen the bond between themselves and their clients; to alleviate the sense of isolation and aloneness that most patients, indeed most people, often experience; and to offer new ways of thinking and acting. In regard to this last point: Sometimes—more often than some therapists realize—clients need concrete suggestions or new models of behaving and feeling. These models may be created through homework assignments or in-session "brainstorming," but may be especially influential when offered through the affectively charged here-and-now medium of therapist disclosure. Knox and Hill (2003) suggested one other important function of therapist disclosure: This behavior encourages patients' own disclosures.

Among the least endorsed reasons for disclosing in the Lane et al. (2001) study, therapists noted their own satisfaction in sharing and being open. These therapists felt they should not act in accord with their own narcissistic needs or at least felt they could not acknowledge having done so. Consistent with this finding, the two most frequently endorsed reasons for not disclosing to a patient were therapists' sense that a given disclosure might interfere with the flow of the patient's material and, similarly, that the disclosure would shift the focus of attention from the patient. In Anderson and Mandell's (1989) survey of 365 practicing social workers, the most common reasons cited for not disclosing was shifting focus from the client, decreasing the time available for client disclosure, interfering with the transference, creating role confusion, and deviating from the client's expectations of professional behavior. Thus, the research indicates that most therapists appropriately assume that their primary task is to focus on the needs of their clients—not their own needs to appear or feel smart, useful, or friendly.

Knox et al. (1997) studied clients' perceptions of therapists' disclosures. Subjects in this study (all in long-term therapy) reported four primary positive effects of these behaviors: They facilitate new perspectives on issues, including new ways of thinking, feeling, or behaving; they serve to make the therapeutic relationship more egalitarian; they provide reassurance that many of their issues are normal universal concerns; and they serve as a model of interpersonal openness that may lead to greater disclosure of their own issues. In addition, according to these clients, helpful therapist disclosures involve sharing personal information, occur when they (clients) are discussing their own important personal issues, and can be seen as attempts by therapists to normalize concerns or provide reassurance. Thus, clients' perceptions of the benefits of therapist self-disclosure correspond closely to therapists' rationales for such disclosures.

That many contemporary therapists seemingly value self-disclosure more than their counterparts of several decades ago is consistent with the tenets of the newer cognitively oriented models that emphasize active collaboration between patient and therapist, and also with newer relationally oriented psychodynamic models that are premised on the idea of a mutually influential and oft-examined "two-person field." Furthermore, as has been noted previously, therapist disclosure is consistent with the general societal trend toward democratization and role informality, even within professional relationships.

EFFECTS OF THERAPIST DISCLOSURE

Existing research on the effects of therapist disclosure has relied primarily on analogue methodology in which simulations of therapy, rather than actual therapy, are evaluated by outside observers. Hill and Knox (2002) reviewed the analogue research and concluded that nonclient observers tend to perceive both therapist self-disclosing and self-involving statements favorably: 14 out of 18 studies reported positive perceptions of therapist self-disclosing statements, and 6 out of 7 studies reported positive perceptions of therapist self-involving statements. Watkins' (1990) earlier extensive review of the analogue research also suggested generally positive effects: Therapists who self-disclose in moderation and in a not-too-intimate way tend to be viewed more favorably and elicit more client self-disclosure than therapists who do not disclose at all, who disclose a great deal, or who disclose personal or intimate material.

Hill and Knox (2002) have pointed out that, whereas analogue research can provide heuristically useful information about the effects of therapist self-disclosure, the information remains limited in its generalizability. Moreover, as Orlinsky and Howard (1986) noted, "real-life" studies of the effects of therapist self-disclosure on therapy outcome have yielded less consistent results than analogue studies. Hill and Knox's review found that most nonanalogue studies have failed to find significant associations between frequency of therapist self-disclosures and client, therapist, or observer judgments of treatment outcome. This, they suggest, is hardly surprising given that these studies have failed to assess the specific nature (e.g., type, manner, or quality) of therapist disclosures.

At least one study (Braswell, Kendall, Braith, Carey, & Vye, 1985) reported a negative relationship between frequency of therapist self-disclosures and therapists' ratings of client improvement. On the other hand, several studies have reported positive effects of therapist disclosure on treatment outcome. For example, one early study by Truax and Carkhuff (1965) demonstrated a significant relationship between therapist transparency—a Rogerian concept most often "translated" as openness but also viewed as a proxy for therapist disclosure—and the patient's level of self-disclosure or self-exploration. In addition, Barrett and Berman (2001) found that therapist self-disclosure was positively related to outcome (more about this study below), and Ramsdell and Ramsdell (1993) found that former clients believed that therapist disclosure had a beneficial effect on their therapy.

Still other studies (e.g., Audet & Everall, 2003; Curtis, Field, Knaan-Kostman, & Mannix, 2004; Wells, 1994) have noted mixed results. For example, in a qualitative study of eight clients in psychotherapy, Wells found that some participants felt that the therapeutic relationship was equalized as a result of their therapist's disclosure and that this empowered them and validated their experience. However, other clients in this study referred to a significant decrease in trust and confidence in their therapists as well as increased inhibition around sharing their response to their therapist's disclosure. Similarly, Audet and Everall's (2003) study found that therapist disclosure had the positive effects of equalizing the relationship and enabling clients to perceive a commonality of experience with another, but also led to a reduction in clients' trust in the therapist's ability to help and a greater likelihood of their feeling critical of their therapist. Recently, Curtis et al. (2004) studied what 75 psychoanalysts found helpful and hurtful in their own analyses. Their findings indicated that a therapist's disclosure of specific aspects of his or her life (i.e., factual self-disclosure) was not significantly correlated with self-perceived change but that disclosure of feelings was positively correlated with change (p. 194).

Do therapists themselves regard their disclosures as either appropriate or effective? Pope et al.'s (1988) survey of therapists indicated that most (59.4%) felt that "using self-disclosure as a therapy technique" was either "good" or "good under most circumstances" (p. 548). As noted earlier, in Hill et al.'s (1988) study, clients rated therapist disclosures as the most helpful of therapist interventions, but therapists themselves assigned self-disclosures their lowest helpfulness ratings, a finding hypothesized by Hill et al. to reflect therapists' feelings of vulnerability. The apparent discrepancy between these sets of findings may be a function of the different response sets: Therapists responding to Pope et al. may have felt they were primarily rating the appropriateness of self-disclosing, whereas those responding to Hill et al. may have felt as if they were rendering a more specific judgment about its effectiveness as an intervention.

Two studies of the effects of therapist disclosure, one performed by Hill's research team and one recent study by Barrett and Berman, merit special attention inasmuch as they have been widely cited and are more methodologically sophisticated than either analogue studies or relatively straightforward surveys.

Hill et al.'s (1989) study divided therapist self-disclosures into four categories: involving (communication of the therapist's feelings or cognitions regarding the client in therapy), disclosing (statements revealing something about the therapist's life), reassuring (disclosures that reinforce or legitimize the patient's experience), and challenging (disclosures that confront the client's perspectives or behavior). Reassuring disclosures were rated as most helpful by clients and therapists. Statements that were both involving and reassuring were also rated as helpful by both therapists and clients. In addition, this study utilized "client experience" (an indication of the client's affective involvement in therapy) as an outcome measure and found that reassuring disclosures led to higher client experiencing than did challenging disclosures. These results not only make clinical sense but also add a much-needed layer of complexity to studies (e.g., Curtis et al., 2004; McCarthy & Betz, 1978; Watkins & Schneider, 1989) that have found self-involving disclosures to be the most helpful to clients. That is, it may not be the self-involving aspect of the disclosure that is beneficial per se, but rather the reassuring, affirming nature of this behavior. Therapists' "positive regard" of patients has often (though not consistently) been associated with good therapeutic outcome (Farber & Lane, 2002).

The Barrett and Berman (2001) study is especially noteworthy in that it employed a quasi-experimental design—systematically varying levels of therapist self-disclosure to assess the effects of amount of disclosure on therapy outcome. In this study, therapists were doctoral students at a university who had completed at least 2 years of clinical training, and clients were adults over 18 who had requested individual therapy at the university training clinic. Each therapist conducted four sessions with each of two clients. With one client, the therapist increased the frequency of reciprocal disclosure (the disclosure of personal information in response to similar client self-disclosures); with the other, the therapist limited his or her reciprocal disclosures. Therapists were trained in making both reciprocal self-disclosures (i.e., for the "increased" condition) and providing non-self-disclosure responses to client self-disclosures (i.e., for the "limited" condition). That the two conditions differed significantly in terms of the frequency of disclosure was confirmed by blind-observer ratings.

Clients in the condition of increased therapist self-disclosure reported lower levels of symptom distress and greater levels of liking the therapist than those in the condition of limited therapist self-disclosure. However, it is also important to note that increased therapist disclosure did not result in increases in either the frequency or intimacy of patient disclosures. In sum, although this study is limited by its exclusive use of "reciprocal" disclosures, an inexperienced therapist sample, and reliance on a four-session course of treatment, the results provide experimentally derived evidence that therapist self-disclosure can be useful in reducing symptom distress and strengthening the therapeutic alliance.

Constantine and Kwan (2003) have pointed out that "much of the existing literature on therapist self-disclosure has been with White or European American individuals" (p. 582). Cross-cultural differences in therapist self-disclosure have been investigated, but in a limited fashion. For example, Wetzel and Wright-Buckley (1988) found that in the context of biracial counseling interviews a reciprocity effect was found only when black therapists interviewed black clients. No reciprocity effect was obtained when white therapists interviewed black clients. And, in a study using Asian American college students as participants in a one-session therapy-like situation, Kim et al. (2003) found no relationship between level of adherence to traditional Asian cultural values (e.g., deference to authority, self-restraint, filial piety) and perceptions of the helpfulness of the self-disclosures of Caucasian student therapists. Clearly, far more research on the effects of ethnicity and race on therapist disclosure is necessary.

THERAPIST DISCLOSURE TO CHILD PATIENTS

Research on self-disclosure to children mirrors the situation with research on multicultural aspects of therapist disclosure. Relative to the body of research on therapist self-disclosure to adult patients, studies focusing on disclosure to child patients have been scant. This is consistent with the history of psychotherapy research, wherein investigations of variables affecting child clients have lagged far behind studies of adults.

In an attempt to partially remedy the lack of research in this area, Capobianco and Farber (2005) investigated therapists' use of factual self-disclosures with child patients ages 5–12. They found that therapists' estimate of their self-disclosures to their child patients was in the low to moderate range: 3.2 on a 7-point scale.

The most frequently endorsed disclosure item in this study was parental status. In addition to being the most frequently disclosed item, parental status was the most frequently solicited item by child patients, and the one most perceived by therapists to advance treatment aims with child patients. Revealing parental status may be the means for child therapists to show their patients that they understand, and have experience with, children. Other items that therapists disclosed relatively frequently included marital status, their own school experiences, pets, personal values, and hobbies.

Therapists in Capobianco and Farber's study reported that, in general, child patients "almost never" ($M = 2.3$) request personal information from them. By comparison, Lane et al. (2001) found that adult patients "sometimes" solicit therapist disclosures ($M = 4.4$). Given that children are often prohibited from asking adults the same questions that adults ask of them, this discrepancy is not surprising. As one participant noted, "Child clients rarely ask these questions. . . . You have to guess that a question is being asked in an oblique way." Somewhat surprisingly, though, therapists rated the usefulness of disclosing the items on this survey to be low ($M = 2.3$, in the "almost never helpful" range). Previous studies with adult patients have found a much higher rate of helpfulness. Lane et al.'s sample of therapists, for example, reported a mean of 4.7 on a similarly anchored 7-point scale.

Scores on all dimensions of disclosure were found to be unrelated to therapist variables, with the exception of theoretical orientation. Consistent with previous literature (e.g., Lane et al., 2001; Simi & Mahalik, 1997), psychodynamic clinicians in this study self-disclosed with child patients less frequently than those espousing a cognitive-behavioral or eclectic orientation. While one might imagine that contemporary psychodynamic therapists would be influenced by relational concepts that emphasize mutuality and thus view disclosure at least as favorably as clinicians adopting other theoretical perspectives, this was not the case. It is possible, of course, that this finding simply reflects the enduring power of tradition within a given theoretical approach.

It is also possible that a study investigating the frequency and perceived helpfulness of self-involving disclosures (i.e., those that reflect therapists' statements of their feelings and reactions) rather than factual disclosures would have elicited a different, and perhaps more favorable, set of reactions from these psychodynamically oriented therapists. It should also be noted, however, that Capobianco and Farber's (2005) study did not take into account client variables such as diagnosis, gender, family background, attachment status, or time in treatment. These factors might well influence a therapist's tendency toward self-disclosure above and beyond theoretical orientation.

The results of this research suggest that therapists do not consider self-disclosure of personal factual information a strong part of their therapeutic repertoire with children. Although cognitive-behavioral and eclectically oriented therapists self-disclosed more often than psychodynamic clinicians, the consensus among therapists was that factual self-disclosure does not, in general, advance treatment aims for child patients. However, further research—especially with an explicit focus on outcome—is needed before one can draw definitive conclusions regarding the usefulness of therapist self-disclosure with children. Current questionnaires are incapable of assessing the full range and meaningfulness of disclosures in child therapy. In addition, as noted above, research in this area needs to investigate the virtually unexplored topic of therapist self-involving statements to children. Therapists' perceptions of the value of these interventions may be significantly different from their perceptions of more standard factual self-disclosures.

Moreover, research has not yet adequately attended to the stylistic differences between disclosures in adult and child therapy. Not only is it likely that factual self-disclosures are more common in adult therapy and self-involving disclosures more common in child therapy, but also in the latter form of treatment therapist self-disclosures are more likely to be expressed in a variety of nonverbal ways. Chethik (2000), for example, relates an incident where, in an attempt to convey to a child patient the therapist's incredulity and demonstrate the irrational nature of the child's fears, the therapist not only spoke about the child's mistaken ideas but also hit his own forehead in disbelief. The child was dealing with guilt stemming from his violent fantasies involving his mother and baby sister; merely being "told" that his thoughts and fantasies cannot cause actual physical damage to his family would not have been adequate. By dramatically acting out his own shock, the therapist disclosed his feelings on the subject.

Nonverbal forms of self-disclosure in clinical work with both children and adults include a wide variety of postures (e.g., the way one sits), gestures (e.g., hand, head, eye, and mouth movements), affective expressions (e.g., laughter, smiles, and frowns), and vocalizations (e.g., the pitch, tone, fluency, and volume of one's voice). However, because the maintenance of a strictly professional (adult) demeanor is less appropriate, and less possible, when working with children, the range of nonverbal expressiveness is often far greater in child clinical work than it is in adult treatment. Stated somewhat differently, the degree of playfulness, spontaneity, creativity, and flexibility demanded of (or allowed) a child therapist implies a greater freedom of personal expression. The problem for researchers is that nonverbal forms of therapist expressiveness and self-disclosure are difficult to operationalize, categorize, and measure. It would not be surprising, then, if future research determined that therapist disclosure in child therapy, while of a different order than that in adult psychotherapy, occurs at comparable or even higher rates and has at least equally potent effects on outcome.

In this regard, several authors (Barish, 2004; Gaines, 2003; Gardner, 1993; Leichtentritt & Schechtman, 1998) have proposed a number of over-lapping benefits of self-disclosure to children: strengthening the therapeutic bond (insofar as children value reciprocity), facilitating therapeutic engagement, and encouraging children's own disclosure. These potential benefits are essentially identical to those identified in therapeutic work with adults. In addition, Gaines has suggested that therapist disclosure to children can promote meaningful play, evoke emotions, help identify disavowed feelings, and modify disparaging self-judgments; with older children and adolescents, therapist disclosure may also help alleviate initial resistance to therapy, promote ego development, and heighten the capacity for self-observation.

Barish (2004) has acknowledged that, while he is typically circumspect in self-disclosing to his adult patients, he is "freely self-disclosing" (p. 271) in his work with children; indeed, he suggests to beginning therapists that they allow themselves the freedom to be animated, playful, and even at times silly. In part, he justifies this by suggesting that, even more than adults, children need active emotional engagement and support. Talking personally to children "establishes the therapist as a noncritical and nonthreatening presence" (p. 274). These qualities, argues Barish, are conveyed to children through liberal use of the therapist's "self," including his or her warmth, friendliness, humor, and personal openness. Despite these apparent benefits, as with all clinical interventions, decisions regarding therapist disclosure must be made on a case-by-case basis, as necessitated by the specific needs of the child client.

LIMITATIONS OF THERAPIST
SELF-DISCLOSURE RESEARCH

Hill and Knox (2002) have pointed out several limitations of therapist disclosure research. They've noted that multiple definitions have been used by investigators, making comparisons among studies particularly difficult. They've also shown that studies have typically focused on frequency of disclosure, implicitly assuming an unlikely linear relationship between this variable and therapeutic outcome: "There is no compelling reason to believe that more disclosures should lead to better outcome. It may even be that therapist self-disclosure yields its positive effects because it typically occurs so infrequently" (p. 261). Hill and Knox have also emphasized that much of this research has been atheoretical. No research, for example, has examined whether therapist disclosure contaminates the transference, as asserted by traditional psychoanalytic theorists.

Finally, these authors have drawn attention to two key methodological problems in the literature: a heavy reliance on analogue methodology and the lack of an ideal method for analyzing the effects of disclosure on outcome. Analogue studies are problematic because they are not "experience-near" and thus have limited applicability to actual therapeutic situations. In essence, they decontextualize a situation in which context exerts a great degree of influence. This is true as well of survey research, where therapists merely report their perceived levels and/or content of disclosure. Indeed, all extant methods of studying therapist self-disclosure seem incapable of capturing the full story. Some researchers have proposed temporal models of client self-disclosure (Farber et al., 2004) that view the consequences of disclosure as changing over time. Other researchers have begun to specify which types of client disclosures lead to which kinds of outcomes (Kahn et al., 2001). Similar innovations are needed in the therapist self-disclosure field.

Although research on therapist disclosure features few methodologically complex studies set in real therapeutic contexts, it must be remembered that this line of inquiry is very much in its infancy. Furthermore, as noted in the beginning of this chapter, whereas definitional and methodological issues pose problems for the field, the existing research has established a link between therapist self-disclosure and positive outcome (Hill & Knox, 2002) that future studies can build upon. The clinical implications of the research findings and theoretical developments in this area will be discussed in the next chapter.

CHAPTER 8

Clinical Perspectives on Therapist Disclosure

> The analyst should be impenetrable to the patient, and like a mirror, reflect nothing but what is shown to him.
>
> —FREUD (1912, p. 18)

> In any genuine meeting, both participants stand equally bared before each other.
>
> —SINGER (1977, p. 181)

The two quotes above exemplify the extreme positions on a hypothetical continuum of what theorists consider appropriate therapist disclosures. The first quote reflects the "official" position assumed by most psychoanalysts for much of the 20th century. The second reflects a far more contemporary stance, albeit one assumedly endorsed by only a small minority of current therapists.

This second stance was popularized and implicitly touted as *the* means of therapeutic improvement in the movie *Good Will Hunting*. Among other details of his life, the therapist, Sean Maguire (Robin Williams), shares the following with his patient (Matt Damon): that his wife has died 2 years ago after a long illness, that he's not seeking another woman, that he remembers the exact day when he "knew" she was the one, and that she suffered from flatulence that woke her during sleep. In the climactic scene, he acknowledges that, like his patient, he too has suffered from physical abuse (at the hands of an alcoholic father). Following this admission, patient and therapist share memories of the specific types of articles (e.g., belts) with which they've been hit. The therapist's insistence at the end of this scene that "it's not your fault" is finally heard by the patient. As they tearfully hug, we are left with the inexorable conclusion that the therapist's willingness to disclose so openly is what made this healing moment possible.

It is likely that most therapists have adopted a position somewhere in the middle of this extreme range. Indeed, as the previous chapters have indicated, therapists vary widely in their stance toward self-disclosure, a function of many factors, including their theoretical orientation, personal comfort with this practice, and experiences in their own therapy and supervision. Their disclosures are also likely to be affected by the norms of the setting where they work (if at a clinic or hospital), the types of patients with whom they work, the goals that they have established in collaboration with specific patients, and their sense of how helpful their disclosures have been in the past. Many of these factors will be elaborated upon later in this chapter.

Moreover, whatever their baseline level of self-disclosure with a given patient, therapists undoubtedly vary the nature of their disclosures in response to their perceptions of what is clinically appropriate at any given time. These moment-to-moment decisions are themselves influenced by myriad variables that typically fall somewhere between background and foreground (or conscious and unconscious), including the gender configuration of the therapeutic dyad, the amount of time left in the session, the current emotional state of the patient, and, arguably most importantly, the therapist's clinical instinct as to how this potential disclosure will be experienced by the patient. Taken together, these factors and perhaps a host of others make the decision to disclose an enormously complicated matter. As Johnston and Farber (1996) showed, most therapists have adopted a flexible attitude toward self disclosure, varying their practice according to the clinical situation at hand.

Although patient and therapist disclosure are often discussed in tandem, therapist disclosure is not the obverse of patient disclosure. They are of a different order and serve very different purposes. Although we can identify some commonalities—for example, both therapist and patient disclosure have been linked to positive therapeutic outcome, and both may lead to increased feelings of authenticity and genuineness—the essential differences are more pronounced. Patients are there to discuss what is on their minds and troubling them, to become known, and to reveal their secrets; none of this is true for therapists.

Patient and therapist disclosure are not even truly complementary phenomena. Ferenczi's failed clinical experiments in the 1930s convinced most therapists of that era that true complementarity and mutuality of disclosure are neither clinically possible nor desirable; this position continues to be predominant in the contemporary psychotherapeutic community. In addition, recent research (Barrett & Berman, 2001) has cast some doubt on long-held assumptions regarding reciprocity effects in therapy, indicating that, at least in those instances when therapist disclosures follow patient disclosures, subsequent patient disclosures do not increase in frequency or intimacy. While this research did not address an equally important hypothesis—the question of whether unsolicited "therapist-first" disclosures encourage subsequent patient disclosures—it does raise questions about the true extent and limits of reciprocity within the treatment setting.

Still, therapist disclosure is important in its own right. For all the reasons noted in Chapter 7—for example, that it affirms and normalizes patient experiences, provides new ways of understanding and behaving, and promotes a deeper therapeutic relationship—disclosure has become an integral aspect of most therapists' work.

This chapter will focus on clinical aspects of therapist self-disclosure—what theorists and therapists have had to say about its nature and value as well as the special circumstances (e.g., therapist pregnancy or illness) that may dictate its use. Taken as a whole, this voluminous literature suggests that clinicians must attempt to reconcile the tension among three competing needs: first, to be as helpful as possible to patients, according patients the substantial benefits of disclosure; second, to respect and adhere to firm professional boundaries that afford a sense of safety and reflect an unwavering commitment to attend to the needs of the patient; and third, to express themselves in a genuine and open manner, one reflecting the profound sense of intimacy or potential intimacy in the relationship. The struggle to balance these needs at any given point in therapy is formidable and often occurs with varying degrees of awareness. Complicating this situation, many writers have suggested that disclosure occurs virtually constantly, regardless of intentionality, and that debate over its use should focus on what, how, and when rather than whether.

ARE THERAPIST DISCLOSURES INEVITABLE?

It is now widely accepted that a therapist cannot truly remain unknown. As suggested earlier, his or her clothing, demeanor, tone of voice, vocabulary, office decor, and body language all provide significant personal information to an observant patient. Singer's (1977) provocative paper "The Fiction of Analytic Anonymity" questioned the assumptions of therapist invisibility by challenging the then-prevailing notion that a therapist's words yielded little or no information about him or her per se. His thesis was that therapists' comments, especially those that are astute, necessarily reveal aspects of the therapist's own history and dynamics. Most patients, he contended, are intuitively aware that "it takes one to know one" and that therapists' ability to understand and provide help inevitably stem from their experience in grappling with similar problems. Of course, from this perspective, virtually everything a therapist says could be considered self-disclosing. And while in some ways this is true—that is, every verbalization necessarily reflects an individual's unique perspective, history, and experience—adopting this view dilutes the more useful if narrow meaning of therapist self-disclosure.

Nevertheless, from Singer's perspective, all forms of clinical intervention involve a certain degree of disclosure: "The structure, focus, and content of the analyst's response to the patient reveals the analyst's private religion, no matter what his pretenses to himself and others" (p. 184). Note the word "pretenses" though—Singer's sense is that therapists, especially analysts, are more aware than they acknowledge publicly that they give themselves away in what they say and how they act with patients. Interpretations serve as a good example. According to Singer, "What analysts so fondly think of as interpretations are neither exclusively nor even primarily comments about their clients' deeper motivations but first and foremost self-revealing remarks" (p. 183). Marcus (1998), among other contemporary therapists, makes much the same point when he suggests that "at some level" patients always know the truth behind their therapists' emotional responses (p. 236). Therapists' reluctance to admit the extent to which their patients get to know them is due to their fear of not being accepted by their patients (Singer) or to their having grown too accustomed to the experience of being idealized (Renik, 1995). According to Singer, the question "Will the patient accept me if he knows me?" is always lurking in the therapist's mind. Thus, Singer took therapists to task for what he regarded as their too frequent failures to act courageously in regard to disclosures—that is, for their reluctance to interpret out of fear that their remarks would reveal all too well that they, too, have "been there," or that their patients would no longer regard them with quite the same degree of respect and awe.

Singer's remarks are in some ways quite important and in other ways somewhat outdated. Importantly, Singer reminds those in the mental health profession that the need to feel larger than life or special is an ongoing occupational hazard that can interfere with good treatment. Indeed, this admonition, in one form or another, has been part of the literature in the field at least since 1913, when Ernest Jones wrote about the "God complex" in therapists. The classic updates on this theme included Marmor's (1953) paper on "feelings of superiority" in psychiatrists and Sharaf and Levinson's (1964) article on therapists' "quest for omnipotence." Singer's variation on this theme—that therapists needn't struggle so hard to avoid being seen and perceived as fallible, especially since this is all but unavoidable anyway—was a significant contribution to the field; indeed, he was among the first to recognize the many ways in which therapists, through their words, invariably become known to their patients. On the other hand, Singer's words are less revolutionary in an age in which relationally oriented therapy has become the dominant motif in psychodynamic circles and the power of the relationship has become a "given" in essentially every form of therapy. Within this newer paradigm, there is far less reluctance for therapists to become known; indeed, there is pressure for the opposite. Therapists as well as patients are likely to acknowledge and explore the mutative influence of the therapists' active presence within the therapeutic dialogue. As Bridges (2001) has remarked: "Self-disclosure is not only an inevitable, but also an essential, aspect of the psychotherapeutic process" (p. 22).

"Simply" through his or her presence, the therapist can convey a great deal of information to a patient. In Geller's (2005b) conception of the therapist's presence, the communication is decidedly nonverbal: "The deepest sources of presence can be found in processes that move through our bodies, and take place, more or less, below the threshold of conscious awareness . . . depth and rate of breath, the shapes taken by micro-movements of the facial muscles, pitch of voice, the stillness of postures, and temperature regulation" (p. 475). For Geller, these qualities can exert a powerful, often unconscious influence within the therapeutic situation—something on the order of nonverbal reciprocity. A therapist's calm presence, for example, may work to induce calmer physiological states within the patient. As the therapist's calmness is transmitted to the patient directly and with "phenomenological 'immediacy'" (p. 475), the patient experiences deepening of breath, muscle relaxation, and other physiological changes. Conversely, we might hypothesize that a therapist's manifest or even subtle anxiety will induce a sense of anxiety in the patient. Geller suggests, and I concur, that given the importance of the atmosphere they help create, therapists should strive toward a greater awareness of the ways in which they express themselves nonverbally.

WHAT ARE THE DILEMMAS UNDERLYING THE DECISION TO DISCLOSE?

Marcus (1998) stated that while the typical position of analysts today is that it is generally best not to disclose thoughts and feelings to the patient, there are times when doing so may prove to be an effective tool in advancing the treatment. Similarly, Wachtel (1993) suggested that the "particular requirements of a given patient at a given moment in the work must guide the therapist's choices" (p. 223). It is hard to argue with these sentiments, but they both beg the very difficult clinical question of how to decide whether and what disclosures are appropriate at any given moment.

At times, the decision to disclose seems relatively straightforward or uncomplicated: A particular disclosure feels clearly helpful to the patient, unthreatening to therapeutic boundaries, and relatively nonnarcissistic. Or, alternatively, a potential disclosure feels minimally beneficial to the patient, somewhat outside typical professional boundaries (e.g., too colloquial, personally intimate, or provocative), and essentially self-gratifying. But these are the easy cases. More difficult choices arise when the potential benefits and risks seem equally balanced. Thus, even when a therapist believes firmly that there are benefits to disclosing, he or she may be legitimately concerned with other considerations: Will my disclosure set up expectations for more frequent and intimate disclosures? Similarly, will my disclosure be perceived as a reward by my patient, such that subsequent nondisclosure (or less intimate disclosure) will be perceived as withholding or punitive? Will my disclosure burden my patient with knowledge that he or she cannot process well? Will my disclosure be perceived as an implicit communication that there was a better way of doing, saying, or thinking about something? Disclosures, after all, even well-meaning ones, may be experienced as critical comments. They may miss the mark or may be perceived by patients as a misattunement, that is, a too blatant attempt to change the way they feel or think (see Stern, 1985).

The thoughtful clinician must also deal with questions related to the limits of permissible self-gratification. That is, to what extent are the personal benefits of self-disclosure (e.g., experiencing a sense of genuineness or mutuality) acceptable either because the patient is also benefiting or because occasional ego gratification is deemed reasonable or even necessary in the context of a positive therapeutic relationship? Many if not most therapists seem to hold to the position that the question behind every self-disclosure should be either "does the disclosure aid in the patient's therapy?" or, similarly, "Is this particular disclosure appropriate for this particular patient?" However, judging from more recent literature, especially that in the humanistic and relational fields, more therapists are now considering how their own needs to experience gratification, intimacy, or authenticity can be legitimate factors in determining their therapeutic stance, including their interactions with patients.

Thus, more therapists are writing and talking about their need to "be in the room" more fully and in a more self-disclosing manner. Still, the opposite position—that of narcissistic temptation—must also be considered. As Basescu (1977) has noted, the practice of psychotherapy contains "so many opportunities and temptations for self-aggrandizement and self-gratification" (p. 155). Finding the right balance between these positions can be difficult even for the most considerate therapist. This may be especially the case for psychoanalysts who, suggests Aron (1991), are often made anxious by the tension between gratifying their patients' desire to know them more deeply and their own desire to remain hidden and relatively anonymous.

Basescu (1977) offers a poignant, courageous discussion of his struggle to reconcile his desire to be helpful, his need to feel fully human and open in the therapeutic relationship, and his wish to avoid fulfilling essentially egotistical needs:

> The whole issue of disclosing myself in my work as a therapist is one that is shot through with nagging anxieties for me because I wonder what my

real intentions are when I answer personal questions or deliberately describe something about myself—an experience, event or feeling—and I wonder about the kind of impact it has on the other person. I know that the conception of the role of the therapist has evolved from that of the anonymous reflector, through that of the participant observer, to the current standard of the therapist as human being. It is not so easy for me to be a human being. I think it would be easier for me to be a mirror. The rules for being a mirror are more clear-cut than the rules for being human. . . . The combination of my awareness of purpose and the feeling I have that being open and "human" is desirable is, I think, what gives rise to my moments of doubt about what is going on when I talk about myself or expose my feelings (or avoid talking about myself).

Am I looking for attention or creating an impression? Am I playing a role? Am I giving in to pressure? Am I cooperating with avoiding something? Am I serving my needs or the other person's? (I realize, incidentally, that serving my needs has its place and therapeutic value in my work, but that doesn't simplify the problem of my doubts. It complicates it.) Am I conveying understanding by describing a similar experience of my own? Am I being reassuring by saying I have experiences like yours? Am I just being me as a way of saying, "It's all right for you to be just yourself" . . . My point is that as the value of self-disclosure by the therapist has become recognized, it has provided me with, among other things, additional opportunities to worry and wonder. It is much easier to avoid all self-disclosure than to have to decide what is or is not desirable to express. But is it more therapeutic? (pp. 159–160)

Another disclosure-related dilemma pertains to therapists' responsibility toward answering patients' direct questions. Here, too, Basescu (1987) challenged the prevailing clinical wisdom. He disputed the logic behind analysts' traditional reluctance to respond to patient requests for information or feedback. This logic grew out of the assumption that patients needed to remain focused exclusively and intently on their own issues and that their interest in their therapists' thoughts or private lives was essentially a form of resistance to exploring their own experiences and fantasies. Basescu, however, averred that the decision to not answer direct questions contributes to the "mystification" of patients' experiences. "I think," said Basescu, "that too often, with the intention of allowing the patient's fantasies and projections free reign, analysts avoid the kind of self-disclosure that can have far greater therapeutic value. Getting direct, open, forthright feedback about the impact one has on others may be one of the important aspects of the therapeutic experience—for both participants" (p. 260). Thus, Basescu acknowledged, "I often ask [patients], What are you thinking?, and I often answer it when it's asked of me" (p. 260). To Basescu, then, and to the increasing number of others (including myself) whose professional development has been infused with an appreciation for the overriding value of the therapeutic relationship, disclosing in direct response to patients' questions offers a propitious opportunity for furthering patients' awareness of their role in relationships and the way they are perceived by important others. Even answering relatively mundane questions may be a means by which therapists allow patients to know that they are important and that their needs will be taken seriously.

An often overlooked but potentially important clinical point: Therapist disclosures are often thought to fall into one of two convenient categories—helpful and harmful. But some disclosures may simply fall flat, go nowhere, land harmlessly on ears that are attuned to matters of greater importance. "Hmm, I saw that movie, too"; "Yes, I do have a bit of a cold"; "I don't watch much TV"—all are disclosures that, to most patients, have little impact. Despite therapists' undoubted importance to patients, every therapist disclosure is not regarded by patients as profound and deserving deep consideration.

Similarly, some disclosures, especially those that are solicited directly by patients, may serve to gratify an immediate need to know something about the therapist or to temporarily shift the dialogue away from the patient, but may not be experienced as especially helpful or harmful. These disclosures may have the salutary effects that Basescu (1987) posited, the negative effects (i.e., therapists' inadvertent collusion with patient resistance) that many have feared, or fall somewhere in the middle in terms of impact. The frequency, content, timing, and tone of these disclosures are all likely to affect the outcome. It is also worth noting that, while some therapist disclosures have little impact on patients, a therapist's failure to disclose requested information or to respond to a patient's need for affirmation or feedback may foster considerable resentment and resistance.

It is also important for therapists to be aware that, while individual acts of self-disclosure may in each instance be appropriate, excessive disclosure may be problematic. Therapists who constantly self-disclose are likely to appear inappropriate and even narcissistic to clients. In recounting her termination from a long-term, mostly helpful, therapeutic relationship, a new patient of mine focused on her sense that her therapist didn't leave her "enough space" in the room; from her perspective, he needed to react to virtually everything she said. In addition, therapists who disclose excessively may also be "setting up" vulnerable clients to believe that they have very special relationships with their therapists. In certain cases, this belief may extend to a hope, wish, or expectation that the relationship expand beyond the boundaries of the therapist's office.

Yet another dilemma: Highly personal factual disclosures, as well as explicitly self-involving disclosures, are often both high-gain and high-risk. "I feel frustrated," "I feel taken advantage of," "I'm aware of the sexual tension in the room," "I care for you a great deal," "I too have felt that way," "Yes, I am married and have two children," "No, I have never experienced the kind of abuse that you did"—are all powerful statements with the potential for strengthening or reestablishing a position of intimacy between patient and therapist. Self-involving disclosures also have the potential for affording patients an awareness of their role in the evocation of powerful (and usually unremarked-upon) interpersonal dynamics. When therapists acknowledge their feelings (e.g., of frustration, confusion, or tenderness) or remark upon the feelings present in the room, they present patients with information that they (the patients) rarely receive from others.

At the same time, these disclosures also have the potential to derail the therapeutic relationship and to feel hurtful. Patients may get frightened by any of several aspects of these types of disclosures: They may fear the intimacy that such disclosures evoke and, in some cases, may experience them as too provocative or potentially sexual; they may become overwhelmed at being confronted with aspects of themselves that they find shameful or, similarly, feel criticized by the therapist's comments; they may feel burdened by the knowledge of certain personal therapist disclosures and may feel obliged to shift their focus to the therapist's experience or issues; they may regard the therapist as excessively narcissistic and too invested in sharing his or her needs, feelings, or stories; they may feel anxious in hearing about a therapist's vulnerabilities or experiences and, as a result, lose trust in the therapeutic process. More generally, patients may not be ready or prepared to work with this kind of material, and may feel that they have not "signed up" to learn about these deep aspects of themselves or their therapists or to be involved in a relationship that involves high degrees of intimacy. The importance of caution and of assessing the ability of patients to benefit from a therapist's disclosure has been highlighted by McWilliams (1994): Therapist self-disclosure, she notes, is essentially "irreversible. . . . One cannot become more 'invisible' again" (p. 76).

Therapists' expressions of sexual attraction to patients are likely to be clinically, ethically, and legally problematic. Even when they are not acted upon, these disclosures typically lead to adverse therapeutic consequences (McNamara, 1994; Pope, Sonne, & Greene, 2006). Moreover, as noted in Chapter 6, sexual encounters in therapy—explicitly prohibited by professional codes of ethics—frequently begin with therapist disclosures of romantic or sexual feelings. Pope et al. (2006) acknowledge that there can be no prohibition against these feelings *per se*. They occur for most therapists and they can hardly be outlawed or even discouraged; an awareness of them may even be clinically useful as awareness of powerful countertransferential feelings often is. Winnicott made the essential point that clinical work suffers when therapists deny strong, shameful feelings (e.g., anger) in his classic 1949 article, *Hate in the Countertransference*. But there is a significant difference between experiencing feelings and disclosing them, and therapists need to keep in mind this fundamental distinction. In addition, there is a significant difference between disclosures of caring and disclosures of physical attraction toward patients. In Pope and Tabachnick's (1993) study of nearly 300 therapists (equally divided between male and female), 94% acknowledged telling a female client that they cared for her, but only 37% reported telling a female client that she was physically attractive. Although it is possible to imagine scenarios where verbal expressions of a patient's attractiveness are not egregiously inappropriate (e.g., when a patient is "all dressed up" for an important event), far more often than not these disclosures (and certainly those that are direct expressions of romantic or sexual attraction) reflect the therapist's needs and not those of his or her patients. As such, they are usually considered boundary violations (Gabbard & Lester, 1995).

Even seemingly benign self-involving disclosures may overwhelm the defenses of vulnerable or shame-prone patients. But with high-risk/high-gain, self-involving disclosures, a great deal of tact is usually necessary with even the most well-functioning patients. Couching these types of observations as possibilities or hypotheses may be helpful: "It feels to me" or "I have the sense that . . . what's your experience?" As Geller (1994) has observed about the process of offering one's candid experience of the therapeutic process to patients: "Great tact, kindness, and something akin to connoisseurship are required of a therapist if he/she is to maximize the therapeutic benefits of familiarizing patients with the dysfunctional consequences of their interpersonal style" (p. 13).

According to Hill and Knox (2002), therapists are aware of the potential misuses and negative consequences of disclosure. "Therapists indicated on surveys that they generally *avoided* self-disclosure when the disclosure would fulfill their own needs, move the focus from the client to the therapists, interfere with the client's flow of material, burden or confuse the client, be intrusive for the client, blur the boundaries between the therapist and client, overstimulate the client, or contaminate the transference" (p. 259, emphasis in original). Undoubtedly, there is a great deal of truth to these findings, and we should be thankful that this is the general state of affairs. But these responses also feel too socially desirable and too devoid of the complexity that is inherent in most clinical situations. As therapists of old were almost surely more active, supportive, advice-giving, and reassuring than stereotypes would predict, my hypothesis here is that in actual clinical situations many contemporary therapists are not quite so bound to these ideals as surveys have indicated. These findings, then, may more accurately reflect therapists' ideal rather than real selves.

WHAT OF SILENCE?

His silence is killing me. Sometimes when I get deep into thought,
I feel that it would not be possible for him—the person who
taught me to open—to devise a more terrible punishment than
total silence. . . . I believe he is intentionally trying to drive me to
suicide.

—Yalom (p. 27)

For the most part, Freud prescribed silence and proscribed disclosure for psychoanalysts. But, as has been consistently noted, the field has moved toward far greater acceptance of therapist disclosure and active therapist participation. Thus, assigning an appropriate clinical place for silence has grown more difficult. Silence and attentiveness no longer seem linked in the imaginations of either therapists or patients. Lengthy silence has become aligned with the more discredited aspects of traditional psychoanalysis, seemingly out of place in contemporary relationally oriented therapy and certainly out of place in the more cognitive-behavioral therapies. Silence seems almost anachronistic, a poor fit with a society that expects openness and intimate disclosures in virtually all dyads.

As far back as the 1950s, Anna Freud considered the use of silence unwise in the treatment of adolescents (it increases already high degrees of resistance), and since then its use with adults has been mocked and widely misunderstood by the media. It has been linked to therapist aloofness, arrogance, authoritarianism, and defensiveness. Cartoons have depicted silent therapists as sleeping or even secretly doing crossword puzzles. Presumably, very few contemporary patients would accept a referral to a therapist whose style was characterized by a high degree of silence.

It is easy to forget that shared silence may be therapeutic and that, paradoxically, a therapist's silence may facilitate a patient's disclosure. "Speaking, in psychoanalysis, has been discussed so much that many people overlook almost entirely the emotional effects of silence" (Reik, 1948, p. 122). "In the majority of cases," noted Reik (a disciple of Freud's), "this silence has a calming, beneficent effect. The patient interprets it preconsciously as a sign of quiet attention, one that in itself gives him proof of sympathy. This silence asks him to speak freely and to suspend conventional inhibitions in his talk during the analytic session" (pp. 123–124). Furthermore, Reik contended that a therapist's silence "makes small talk transparent and has a force that pulls the patient forward, driving him into deeper layers than he intended" (p. 123–124). In fact, thought Reik, the silence of the therapist "works even more strongly than words could" (p. 124). Thus, if Reik (and many like-minded classical psychoanalysts) are correct, one of the primary effects of a therapist's silence is to close up the discrepancy between what patients speak of and what is truly salient to them—an omnipresent problem in most therapies. In the throes of a therapist's silence, patients become more aware of what truly is and is not important to discuss. Silence is profound and powerful; in its purest form it endows patients with enormous respect for the formidable task that faces them. In Carlyle's words, "Speech is of time; silence is of eternity" (cited in Reik, 1948, p. 125).

Thus, another question to consider: When is silence a better therapeutic choice than disclosure (or any one of a number of other clinical interventions)? Or, a related question with special relevance to contemporary practice: What is the place of silence in psychotherapy? After all, empathy has largely replaced silence in humanistic/existential psychotherapies, disclosure has largely replaced silence in contemporary psychodynamic therapies, and confrontation has largely replaced silence in short-term dynamic therapy. Why then would a clinician ever be silent? While there can be no definitive rules here, two guidelines may be useful: First, silence is often a good option when the therapist senses that the patient has not finished a thought, idea, or narrative account and that resistance is only minimal. That is, the therapist has a feeling that the resistance does not have to be met "head on" and that, instead, a period of respectful silence may elicit greater patient responsiveness. Second, silence may be indicated in those instances when the therapist has nothing particularly useful to offer. As one of my early supervisors (circa 1976) once said to me: "Just don't say something, sit there."

Nonetheless, silence, like disclosure, has its dangers and may be easily misinterpreted; this seems to be especially true now since silence may no longer signify softness, patience, and attentiveness. Thus, silence should now ideally be used when there seems to be a strong likelihood that it will be interpreted by both parties as "I'm gently waiting, I know there's more, please proceed at your own pace without my interruption." Otherwise, consistent with what Carl Rogers used to do with some regularity, a simple empathic "I know this is difficult" followed by silence may well be a better option. What comes to mind here, too, is Winnicott's deceptively simple statement to his patient: "I've nothing particular to say yet, but if I don't say something, you may begin to feel I'm not here" (cited in Guntrip, 1975, p. 153). Gifted therapists from very different traditions have always been aware of the need for flexibility in the face of the particular needs of a particular patient at a particular time. Both Winnicott and Rogers understood well that at times therapeutic silence could feel quite frightening.

WHAT ARE THE CONSEQUENCES OF NONDISCLOSURE?

To be sure, therapist disclosures and silence do not constitute the universe of alternatives available to therapists in the course of a session. But even as Reik and some contemporary psychoanalysts (e.g., Langs) have cautioned against the excessive use of therapist disclosures, other contemporary therapists have cautioned against their restricted use. Among others, Safran and Muran (2000) have suggested that the withholding of self-involving therapist disclosures can impede the progress of therapy. Fosha (2004) recently provided a lyrical description of how this could occur:

> I have found that when my feeling is that I want to share something with a patient, but then don't, i.e., when the internal thrust of my experience is

naturally forward, but I stop it for whatever reason, be it shyness/personal reticence, or technical, or submission to the internalized pressures of a more neutral way of working, what have you—then it has at times had a negative effect on the flow of the session. It is like damming up the natural flow of dyadic resonance and action tendencies and the process somehow suffers. When I have gone with precisely those internal tendencies, the therapy has usually both soared and deepened.

Both therapists and patients may become frustrated when therapists hold back their thoughts or feelings. Patients are deprived of what may well be useful feedback. As noted earlier, many benefit more from explicit, assumedly objective, immediate feedback about how they come across to others than to the slow accrual of self-insight. Moreover, therapists who are reluctant to make their views and feelings known deprive patients of appropriate models of disclosing risky material. When therapists fail to express their frustration or needs, they make it even more difficult for patients to express directly their negative feelings about their therapist—a common pattern of concealment (Hill et al., 1993).

The inability to speak about difficult feelings, according to Geller (1994), occurs when either member of the therapeutic dyad attempts to "anxiously avoid the burdens of making choices and taking actions that might induce shame or guilt in one or both participants" (p. 15). While it is easy to appreciate the caution and tact exhibited in such situations, it is also important to realize that avoiding mention of the conflictual parts of a relationship may limit expression and growth. Thus, according to Geller, "Stalemated therapies may arise because of the vicious cycles set in motion by mutual withdrawal from the risks of truth-telling" (p. 15). In turn, stalemated therapies may lead to the mutual experience of boredom. Geller has also speculated that the inability to discuss "delicate issues" with a patient may be especially shameful and distressing to those therapists who regard authenticity as a prime virtue. We may wonder, too, whether therapists' reticence in making their views known within sessions contributes to patients' decisions to prematurely terminate therapy.

WHAT FACTORS INFLUENCE THERAPIST DISCLOSURE?

Of all the variables potentially affecting therapist self-disclosure, theoretical orientation has been most widely addressed in the literature. As has been noted, therapists in the classic psychoanalytic tradition have limited their self-disclosure, contending that it interferes with the development of the transference. Those adhering to this position also tend to assert that the therapist's nonwavering empathic interest allows the patient to express feelings freely without the concerns typical of normal "give-and-take" social interaction; that even brief and temporary reversal of roles may place undue burdens on the patient; that the patient's disclosures might be constrained if he or she perceives the therapist's feelings or behavior as a more acceptable standard; and that a precedent for self-disclosing could be set for the future in contexts where it would be less appropriate (Gabbard & Lester, 1995; Langs, 1974, 1978, 1984; Mathews, 1989; Wells, 1994).

As discussed in the preceding two chapters, therapists influenced by other theoretical perspectives have generally espoused very different views of disclosure. To briefly reiterate: For therapists aligned with the various relational schools of contemporary psychoanalysis, disclosure is an inextricable aspect of the mutuality and cocreation of meaning that serve as the bases for instructive observation and healing (e.g., Goldstein, 1994, 1997; Renik, 1995, 1999, 2002). Those therapists influenced by the work of Carl Rogers also tend to be favorably disposed toward therapist disclosure. Rogers (1957) argued that therapist genuineness, a characteristic that includes disclosing personal information when appropriate, is instrumental in fostering client growth and effective therapist–client relationships. Similarly, therapists practicing within an existential framework have traditionally advocated frank therapist disclosure. Yalom (2002), for example, contends that "there is every reason to reveal oneself to the patient and no good reason for concealment" (p. 83). Even cognitive-behavioral therapists, once so wedded to technical as opposed to relational interventions, have begun to accept the mutative aspects of therapist disclosure. Goldfried et al. (2003), for example, have posited that disclosure can be an effective tool in cognitive-behavioral therapy because it can serve to enhance therapeutic techniques (e.g., reinforcement, modeling) that are central to this orientation.

Another therapist factor that may affect the tendency toward disclosure is therapist experience level. Although Simon's (1990) study indicated that experience does not affect frequency of disclosures, a good deal of clinical evidence suggests that this variable may influence the type and process of disclosures. For example, as a way of controlling anxiety, some inexperienced therapists may hold tightly to perceived "rules" and avoid disclosing anything remotely personal. Others may reveal personal aspects of themselves out of a need to establish a nonhierarchical, informal therapeutic relationship while experiencing great difficulty in offering self-involving process-oriented disclosures. Geller (1994) has suggested that "young and relatively inexperienced therapists who feel insecure . . . anxiously avoid confronting patients with those aspects of their self-presentation that may repel interest" (p. 8). Yet another potentially influential therapist variable is that of personal comfort. Some therapists are simply more comfortable than others with the connection, tension, tone, and affect (including shame) that their disclosures create in the room. Some may even rationalize their clinical style, including self-disclosures, by invoking post hoc theoretical justifications.

The setting of a practice may also radically influence the nature of therapist disclosure. Therapists with private or institutional office practices are far less visible than are those who see patients in their homes. In the latter case, patients are privy to a wide variety of what might be considered private information, including data about home furnishings, cars, neighbors, and often at least some knowledge about the therapist's family. I practice therapy primarily in my suburban home, and, although there is a separate entrance to the back of my house (one leading directly to a waiting room), over the years many of my patients have inadvertently met my wife (while she was parking her car in front of the house), seen my children (especially my son, who'd often be playing basketball in the driveway), met my dog (who sometimes wandered downstairs past a not completely closed door), dealt with flooding in my basement (adjacent to my office), and encountered various plumbers, carpenters, gardeners, and housekeepers. They know the cars I've driven, the books I've read (many are shelved in the waiting room), the music I listen to (via the CDs lying next to the computer in my office), and, despite reasonably expensive soundproofing, have heard family fights. All these have been discussable, and virtually all to good advantage, even those occurrences of overheard family fighting. Patients can and do profit from an awareness that therapists' lives are not stress-free and that they, too, must deal with the usual vicissitudes of everyday life.

Yet another factor affecting disclosure is the relationship the therapist has with the specific disorder he or she is treating. That is, some therapists have "been there" in terms of alcohol or drug abuse or childhood victimization and may feel especially inclined to disclose this information to a patient who is dealing with similar experiences. In fact, at some settings (e.g., residential treatment centers for eating disorders or drug or alcohol problems), most staff members have had experience with these problems; choosing to work there is often tantamount to a disclosure of their own prior treatment history. Costin and Johnson (2002) indicated that clinicians who have recovered from an eating disorder and who treat patients suffering from the same disorder are often better able than others to model recovery, develop rapport, and challenge patient self-centeredness and denial. However, according to several authors (Costin & Johnson, 2002; McGovern & Armstrong, 1987), therapists' open acknowledgment of their own recovery experiences may also lead to their overidentification with patients and their assumption of responsibility for patients' recovery out of a "sense of mission," thus putting themselves at risk for relapse. In addition, the therapist in this position may not listen attentively to patients' disclosures because of the mistaken assumption that he or she already knows all about it, that is, knows how the patient thinks and feels.

Patient variables are also likely to affect therapists' willingness to disclose and the consequences of such disclosures. Dixon et al. (2001), for example, averred that therapist self-disclosure is most likely to be effective with patients who are either very young or very old, those that expect high disclosure from the therapist, those from a highly expressive culture, and those who exhibit concrete thinking. These patients, according to the authors, would be most amenable to the tangible feedback and alternative perspectives provided by a therapist's disclosure.

McWilliams (1994), author of three highly popular texts on the practice of contemporary psychodynamic therapy, takes a surprisingly conservative stand in regard to therapist disclosure. While touting its use with highly disturbed individuals—"Psychotic-level people require much more emotional self-disclosure than other patients, and without it they will only stew in their own fantasies" (p. 73)—she concurs with traditional admonitions in terms of its use with other patients. "With healthier people, one avoids emotional revelations so that the patient can notice and explore what his or her fantasies are about the therapist's affective state" (p. 73). Thus, she is "quite self disclosing" with psychotic-level individuals: "I have been known to talk about my family, my personal history, even my opinions—anything to put the person at ease with me as an ordinary human being" (p. 75); by contrast, she prefers to remain "carefully opaque" with less disturbed patients.

TWO CLINICAL EXAMPLES

This first example of a therapist disclosure and its consequences is based loosely on a case I supervised. Some of the salient characteristics of both the student and her patient have been changed.

> The patient, KG, was a 30-year-old single white female with a history of familial physical and sexual abuse. Prior to the treatment under discussion, she had been in therapy several times. The therapist was a white fourth-year doctoral student in a psychodynamically oriented PhD program. The first few sessions of this therapy apparently went well, and a positive therapeutic alliance had been formed. In this session, KG began speaking about her progress in therapy, expressing particular pride in having been able to speak assertively to her mother. When asked by the therapist what led her to being able to speak this way, she veered off the topic and abruptly asked, "How old are you?" The therapist replied by telling KG that her question was important and that she would answer it, but that it would be helpful to first explore KG's motivation for asking and her fantasies surrounding the issue. KG was immediately resistant to this approach and replied that

she did not understand why her question couldn't just be answered. The therapist reiterated that she would, in fact, answer the question but felt that they should explore the question first. Again, KG replied vehemently, with hostility and disbelief, that she did not understand why her question just couldn't be answered.

The therapist then explained the therapeutic value of exploring the underlying meaning and fantasies about things that might not seem obvious. KG, however, insisted that the therapist "stop therapizing her," going on to state, "I know what you're doing, but I don't think this therapist stuff is going to work on me. If you don't want to tell me, then don't." In response to this, the therapist said that she could imagine how frustrating this must be for her to not get what she needs immediately, especially since she had experienced significant deprivation in her past.

The therapist went on to say that she understood that KG probably expected her to be helpful, and that by not getting what she expected she might in fact feel "abused." KG replied: "This is just what my previous therapist did all the time, and we got nowhere. I have been through 10 years of 12-step programs and all sorts of therapy, and I know this process. If you had done what you're doing right now 5 years ago, I would have said, 'OK, let's explore it.' But now, I need to know a few things. I need to know who you are so that I can be certain that you can help me. I could tell that my former therapist was from an alcoholic family and that he wouldn't be helpful to me." The therapist then asked whether her being able to help or not was contingent upon her (the therapist's) having had similar experiences. KG responded that it was. Trying to be empathic, the therapist replied, "If I have been through similar experiences, and have been able to help myself, then you would have proof that I would be able to help you." KG answered, "Yes," but then became exasperated and exclaimed: "I just don't know why you can't tell me how old you are!"

At this point, the therapist felt herself growing defensive and experienced the presence of multiple internalized voices. The strongest voice, at least initially, was that of a former supervisor saying, "You give too soon to your patients and in doing so disrupt the development of the transference. Stick to your guns." But she also heard her own "internal supervisor" saying, "No, it's OK to do this, it's important for this patient now and is important for our relationship." She trusted her instincts:

"I'm 29."

"Cool."

"I'm currently a fourth-year doctoral student in the clinical psychology program."

(Pause.) "You don't have to tell me anything if you don't feel comfortable."

(The therapist thinks, "Huh?" and "Who's the therapist here?")
"I do feel comfortable answering. I have no history of alcoholism or abuse in my family. There is some history of eating disorders [one of KG's other issues], but I don't feel it'd be appropriate for me to discuss that in detail."

"Cool, that's great. That's fine."

(Another pause. KG sighs. She is apparently relieved. The therapist sighs and is apparently relieved. The therapist is aware of a strong moment of bonding—KG has maintained strong eye contact and is smiling softly.)

KG asks, "So, what do you want to know? You said you had a few questions for me?"

Undoubtedly, this degree of disclosure would be strongly disapproved of by classical analysts and also perhaps by others who would contend that this therapist went unnecessarily far in her disclosures and that she should have stopped after acknowledging her age. But this example illustrates most strongly the complexity of such decisions—how difficult it is to come up with a rule, or even a decision matrix, that could guide therapists in these situations. My decision would likely have been to have said something on the order of "I'll tell you my age in a moment, but I'd also like to find out why it's important to you"—gratifying the patient's need to know but at the same time reinforcing the notion of the clinical situation as one in which exploring the patient's thoughts, fantasies, and feelings is not only allowed but paramount. But only this student therapist was there in the moment, and only she was privy to the tone and importance of the patient's need to know, and only she had the immediate sense of the beneficial consequences of disclosing even more than the patient had explicitly asked for. Perhaps other, less disclosing, revelations might also have worked—and perhaps the decision to not disclose at all would have ultimately proven therapeutic—but it's also instructive to consider that a whole range of disclosures, some at the very high end of the continuum, can effect positive changes in the relationship and therapy. Finally, this example reminds us that so-called factual disclosures may also be quite intimate and of the high-risk, high-gain variety.

The second example of a therapist disclosure is from a case of an experienced therapist (Fosha, 2004)—again, the gender configuration is a female therapist working with a female patient. The patient, described as a hard-working college student struggling to make sense of a long-standing but unfulfilling relationship, began speaking in one session about her ways of relaxing. Specifically, she began to talk about having her fingernails painted, adding details about which color she preferred and which salon she frequented, and how often she felt she could indulge herself. As Fosha explains:

> "Everything in me was straining to respond, given my own struggle with those kinds of matters, as well as with the feeling of supreme silliness that I was spending mental energy on such matters. This I knew was also my patient's experience . . . I was feeling 'just how trivial can I possibly get?' and was inclined to go past it to something more substantive. Then the patient said something about my fingernails, and I could no longer resist: Off we went on about 3–4 minutes of girl talk, sharing our trials and tribulations about nails and hair . . . it was a very satisfying conversation. It is difficult to capture the energy which this exchange generated, how it catapulted defensive walls within the patient and between us, and led to an incredible deepening. No technique I could possibly think of would ever have achieved such results within a few minutes."

Here again, the benefit of disclosure is manifest in its ability to strengthen the bond between patient and therapist. A greater sense of intimacy ensues following the therapist's disclosure, and there is an intimation that the patient will be able to disclose more deeply following this exchange. We sense that the patient feels she is cared about—she is being taken seriously. Indeed, the power imbalance has been somewhat equalized. What makes this example somewhat unusual is that the disclosed material is manifestly superficial. Sometimes, then, the potency of a therapist's disclosure lies not in the profundity of the material per se but rather in the connection that even seemingly trivial disclosures may evoke.

THERAPIST DISCLOSURES: WHICH, WHEN, AND HOW?

Although there seems to be an emerging consensus in the field that therapist disclosures are not the toxic stuff they were once considered and that they are likely to be far more beneficial than deleterious to the process of therapy, it is still a daunting task for any therapist to determine whether and when specific disclosures are judicious or helpful. In this regard, Barrett and Berman (2001) cautioned that different types of therapist disclosures—for example, self-involving versus factual or spontaneous versus reciprocal—were likely to have a differential impact on patients. In fact, therapists are likely to employ different criteria in deciding whether and when to use each of these forms of self-disclosure.

In a series of articles, Hill and colleagues (Hill, 1989; Hill & Knox, 2002; Knox & Hill, 2003; Knox et al., 1997) have empirically investigated therapist disclosures, reviewed the literature, and, most relevant to this discussion, developed a series of research-based suggestions for practitioners. Their most recent effort (Knox & Hill, 2003) enumerated 10 recommendations for the use of therapist disclosure. What follows is an annotated summary of these recommendations:

• *Disclose, but do so infrequency and judiciously.* Why disclose? Because the research suggests disclosures, especially reassuring disclosures, are helpful. Why infrequently? Because, as has been noted previously in these pages, the very potency of this intervention may be a function of its low frequency of use. Moreover, according to Knox and Hill (2003), "Therapists who never disclose may be experienced . . . as distant, aloof, and impenetrable, and as a result, the therapy relationship may be compromised. In contrast, therapists who disclose too frequently may be experienced as having tenuous therapy boundaries wherein the focus shifts away from the client" (p. 533). Still, there are those, including Yalom (2002), who essentially contend that too much of a good thing is never enough: "I have never had the experience of disclosing too much" (p. 90).

• *Be mindful of the content of what you disclose.* Clearly, certain disclosures are dangerous and virtually always off-bounds (e.g., sexual practices and fantasies). The authors suggest that the most benign, least intrusive disclosures are those that offer straightforward biographical data. Other authors, though (e.g., Geller & Farber, 1997; Safran & Muran, 2000), contend that disclosures that acknowledge the therapist's own mistakes and lapses are especially important in renewing and strengthening the therapeutic relationship.

• *Be mindful of the intimacy level at which you disclose.* Knox and Hill's (2003) suggestion here reflects their sense that "revelations that are too personal may frighten or burden clients, or may be indicative of boundary problems in the therapy relationship" (p. 534). On the other hand, they caution that disclosures that aren't at least somewhat intimate and personal may feel meaningless to clients and achieve no impact.

• *Tailor disclosures to individual clients' needs.* Consistent with almost all theorists writing on this subject, Knox and Hill suggest that different types of disclosures are likely to work better with different types of clients. For example, the literature on clinical work with borderline patients often cautions therapists from revealing too much personal information, noting these patients' penchant for testing the boundaries and using personal information to manipulate the clinical process.

• *Be sure of why you're disclosing.* Echoing the sentiments of many theorists, Knox and Hill aver that therapists should disclose only if they are clear that they are doing so in the service of their clients' needs. However, in recent years more clinicians have contended that there is a legitimate place in therapy for clinicians' needs, including their need to feel genuine in the relationship. Thus, despite what seems to be a prudent, noncontroversial recommendation, the notion that therapists should disclose only for the sake of the client becomes more complicated when therapists' needs become part of the equation. Indeed, it may be quite difficult at times to determine the extent to which each member of the dyad is or isn't benefiting from a therapist's disclosure. Complicating this even further, these benefits may be different at different times—that is, the effects of disclosure may feel different (to both therapist and patient) in the immediate aftermath of a disclosure than several days or weeks or months later.

• *Resume the focus on the client as soon as possible following a disclosure.* Again, the message here is that the appropriate focus of the work is the client and that therapists should avoid giving any other impression. Therapy, according to this view, is not a typical dyadic relationship in which there are equal "turns" and balanced disclosures. Thus, while therapists may be momentarily "genuine," their work and their words must be primarily in the service of their clients.

• *Consider "immediate," self-involving disclosures.* Consistent with discussion earlier in this chapter of high-risk, high-gain disclosures, Knox and Hill (2003) acknowledge the potential benefits of disclosures that focus on "process," that is, on therapists' feelings about what is happening in the room in the moment. The knowledge gained by such disclosures may help the client become aware not only of his or her role in this dyad but, assumedly, in other relationships as well.

• *Consider disclosures in the termination phase of therapy.* This recommendation is based on the authors' sense that it is especially during the termination phase that clients may benefit from perceiving their therapist as genuine and authentic—qualities that therapist disclosures may facilitate. Moreover, they suggest that these personal disclosures and the ensuing benefits may increase the likelihood that clients will continue to do the work of therapy following termination, that is, that clients will more effectively internalize the benign qualities of their therapist (Geller & Farber, 1993).

• *Monitor clients' reactions to disclosures.* Again, this is consistent with points made earlier in this chapter: that it is important, especially with self-involving disclosures, to ask clients how they feel about what has just been said. It is too easy for all of us to misinterpret a personally revealing message or the motives behind it, and this tendency is certainly exacerbated in the highly charged atmosphere of therapy.

• *Disclose on those issues that you have made peace with personally.* The rationale here is that disclosures about unresolved personal issues may too often have the feel of a therapist using the client's therapy as an opportunity to continue his or her own treatment. Moreover, according to Knox and Hill (2003), disclosures on such issues are unlikely to be helpful—therapists in such situations lack sufficient objectivity or distance to provide helpful models. While this recommendation seems prudent, it is also somewhat contrary to the tradition of 12-step programs wherein the counselors themselves are coping with ongoing struggles to maintain sobriety. Of course, it is fair to note that in such cases these counselors have assumedly gone beyond most other survivors in terms of their understanding and mastery of this problem, even if they have not entirely resolved the issue.

These suggestions, while of significant clinical value, must be understood in the context of a field that has only recently begun empirical research into many of its enormously complex issues. Moreover, as many have observed, it is nearly impossible to offer precise rules about when or how therapists should open up or share their experience directly with patients. So much depends on moment-to-moment interactions that cannot be anticipated or categorized.

SPECIAL CIRCUMSTANCES AFFECTING DISCLOSURE

Certain personal events in the therapist's life, or aspects of his or her lifestyle, inevitably affect the nature and process of disclosure. Some, like pregnancy and obvious physical disability, become de facto disclosures—they are manifestly public and visibly "intrude" into the patient's world. Others are somewhat less obvious but visible to a reasonably observant patient, for example, a new engagement ring, the absence of a once-worn wedding band, weight gain, or a different hairstyle. Still others, such as the therapist's sexual orientation or experience with alcoholism or substance abuse, are not generally observable but often press for disclosure in clinical work with patients confronting these same issues. In this section, I focus on the ways in which therapist pregnancy, sexual orientation, and serious illness affect disclosure and its aftermath.

Therapist Pregnancy

The secret of a therapist's pregnancy need not be verbally disclosed; visual disclosure becomes inevitable as the pregnancy progresses. The therapist may feel as though "the balance between her professional and private life is 'unmasked' by this event" (Rosenthal, 1990, p. 213). For the most part, then, pregnancy poses no real choice between disclosure and discretion; rather, the choice is limited to the timing and the style of disclosure. Nevertheless, traditional psychoanalytic guidelines directed pregnant therapists to wait for patients to notice and comment upon the pregnancy, a strategy consistent with the dictum to keep one's private life as distant and separate as possible from therapeutic sessions. For therapists who may themselves feel uneasy or uncomfortable discussing their pregnancy, this tack may aid them in subconsciously (or even consciously) colluding with their patients' denial (Rosenthal).

The temptation for patients and therapists to minimize, sanitize, or even deny a therapist's pregnancy is in part the result of two of its "shameful," difficult-to-discuss aspects: overt body changes (e.g., increased breast size, weight gain) and, relatedly, the undeniable link of pregnancy to sexuality. There is no escaping the fact that pregnancy is a direct, visible expression of sexuality. The therapist's pregnancy is a conspicuous disclosure, albeit a nonverbal one, of her sexual activity. More than one colleague has acknowledged remembering a fear that some of her patients were calculating the day of conception; included in these thoughts was the sense that some patients—especially men with whom there had already been some experience of erotic tension—were also imagining the act itself. Pregnancy, then, like one's sexuality, begins to feel like a very private matter.

Other factors may add to the difficulty of therapist disclosure of pregnancy. For example, the pregnant therapist may be especially aware of her own vulnerability as well as that of her fetus. As several women therapists I know have remarked, the joys of pregnancy do not eliminate its proverbial difficulties, anxieties, and burdens. (These women also noted that it was surprising that these difficulties, especially the physical ones, seemed to be absent from the accounts of pregnant therapists in the professional literature.) Pregnancy, in some ways, mimics physical illness; it is associated with discomfort, nausea, and invasive medical procedures. The fact that these experiences usually culminate in new life, rather than in death, does not entirely erase these physical realities. In this regard, too, a rarely acknowledged reality of pregnancy, especially first pregnancy, is the frequency of miscarriage; mixed with the hopeful and happy expectations of life are significant fears. An event that could lead to one of the greatest joys in life is inextricably bound with the possibility of tragedy. Taken together, the experience of all these emotional and physical stressors may feel overwhelming, leading to the temptation to avoid any discussion whatsoever of pregnancy.

Patients often struggle with the awareness of their therapist's pregnancy, and this too creates awkwardness in the relationship and inhibits open discussion. Reactions to a therapist's pregnancy may be hampered by the gulf between acceptable, socially appropriate responses (e.g., extending congratulations; displaying enthusiasm; adopting a solicitous attitude) and the possibly negative feelings aroused (e.g., fears of abandonment; awareness of envy; experience of rivalry with the growing fetus; doubts about the therapist's dedication to her work; even betrayal). In a "pronatalist" culture, the expression of such negative emotions is especially difficult (Clarkson, 1980). Thus, social norms may obscure the more complex (and often, less positive) patient reactions to pregnancy, and the therapist may have to skillfully probe beneath the "pronatalist facade" to discover the patient's hidden emotions.

A patient's reluctance to express the full range of emotions elicited by the therapist's pregnancy may also stem from an increased perception of the therapist as vulnerable or weak, and thus less able to tolerate anger and negative affect in her patients. To make these matters even more complex, many pregnant therapists have reported that they do indeed experience increased feelings of vulnerability and a desire to shield or protect themselves and their unborn babies from the rage or hostility of their patients.

There is a threat of role reversal when the therapist is perceived as weak, needy, or vulnerable, and the desire to avoid such a reversal may provide a further impetus for denial on both sides. This creates a situation in which it is all too tempting for the therapist to collude with the patient in denying her pregnancy or, after disclosing it, to avoid discussion of difficult feelings, especially her own.

These factors may help explain the phenomenon of patients who are seemingly unaware of their therapist's pregnancy through most of her term. I noted earlier Freud's (1905) observation that "he that has eyes to see and ears to hear may convince himself that no mortal can keep a secret" (p. 215); however, not all those who possess eyes and ears choose to use them to see and hear. In anecdotal accounts by pregnant therapists, some patients' refusal to notice or acknowledge the pregnancy reaches extraordinary peaks of willful blindness. Even therapist attempts to help the patient see, such as through partial or nonverbal disclosures (e.g., wearing maternity clothes) may fail to be noticed. Haber (1992) recounts the tale of a patient, herself a pregnant therapist struggling with issues of disclosure to patients, who remained oblivious to her therapist's pregnancy until the ninth month.

Opposing these factors that serve to inhibit disclosure of therapist pregnancy is the fact that the rules of engagement in most forms of psychotherapy have changed considerably over the past few decades. Pregnancy is now regarded by many contemporary therapists as an opportunity—an especially powerful one at that—to deepen discussion of intense intrapsychic and interpersonal issues. Sexuality, procreation, parenting, oedipal issues, and sibling rivalry are among the profound issues often activated by the stimulus of the therapist's pregnancy (McGarty, 1988). Discussion of a therapist's pregnancy may also lead to the discovery of new, sometimes crucially important, patient information, including past abortions, miscarriages, infertility, and birth of siblings during childhood. An opportunity exists also to deepen the exploration of topics already being addressed in therapy—for example, issues of separation and abandonment.

Thus, despite the anxiety involved, many therapists do disclose their pregnancies and do invite inquiry or discussions around it. Indeed, serious questions regarding the desirability of concealing one's pregnancy for as long as possible, or of waiting till the patient notices the change, have been raised. Patients may not see (or refuse to acknowledge) the pregnancy until the very end, which may not leave enough time to address the meaning of the pregnancy and all its related issues. Moreover, not revealing a pregnancy until relatively late may not provide sufficient time to discuss several important clinical exigencies, including setting beginning and end dates for temporary termination during the therapist's maternity leave and making arrangements for emergency or interim care for the patient. Inadequate preparation may contribute to the regrettable fact that many transferred patients of therapists on maternity leave do not remain in treatment (Chiaramonte, 1986).

The available literature on this topic (mostly limited to individual accounts by pregnant therapists) suggests that there may be certain patient populations for whom working with a pregnant therapist may be contraindicated. Patients with eating disorders, borderline personality disorder, and those seeking abortion counseling are all especially vulnerable to issues raised by pregnancy. These patients appear to be more likely than others to terminate therapy prematurely when the therapist's pregnancy is disclosed (Fuller Stockman & Green-Emrich, 1994). On the other hand, some eating-disordered patients may derive great benefits from the opportunities provided by the therapist's pregnancy—in particular, the chance to work on issues of body image, sexuality, physical maturity, and parenthood (Fuller Stockman & Green-Emrich, 1994). Other populations may also derive particular benefits from treatment with a pregnant therapist—most notably, pregnant women (Al-Mateen, 1991). The therapist's pregnancy may provide a powerful stimulus for positive identification and opportunities to discuss the many issues surrounding pregnancy and childbirth.

Therapist Sexual Orientation

Should a therapist disclose his or her sexual orientation? This issue has been discussed primarily in the context of treatments in which one member of the therapeutic dyad is gay or lesbian and the other is not. Like "whiteness" or physical health, the traditional assumption in the mental health field is that sexual orientation need not be addressed if both participants fall in the statistically "normative" category, that is, white, nondisabled, and heterosexual. This assumption has been increasingly challenged in recent years by proponents of culturally sensitive counseling, who claim that race and sexual orientation are therapeutically important issues even when both therapist and client share the same characteristic. Nevertheless, the literature in the field continues to focus on how these issues play out when there are differences.

The implications of a therapist's nondisclosure of personal sexual orientation may be profound for a gay patient. Particularly in cases where a patient struggles with issues of coming out and societal pressures to remain in the closet, a refusal by the therapist to openly admit or acknowledge his or her sexual identity may be perceived as further discouraging the patient's own disclosure of gay identity (Taylor, 1993). This implicit discouragement may spread beyond the therapeutic setting and into other areas of the patient's life. If the patient suspects or assumes that the therapist is gay, failure to disclose this may well be construed as further evidence that a gay identity is shameful and should be kept hidden, even in one-on-one personal interactions. If the patient assumes the therapist is straight, fears and assumptions about possible homophobic attitudes or of the ability of a straight therapist to understand and empathize with a gay patient may be compounded by nondisclosure.

Similarly, Cerbone (1991) spoke of the need to loosen the concept of therapeutic neutrality when working with gay and lesbian patients, of allowing such patients to learn more about the therapist's attitudes, values, and opinions. Not making such disclosures may be tantamount to pointedly ignoring the negative effects of cultural biases on the patient. My own sense is that, as with all patients who are otherwise different from ourselves, therapeutic silence in response to issues of sexual orientation may be misconstrued by patients as indifference, insensitivity, or disapproval.

Silverman (2001) suggests that there is a difference between hiding something from a patient and choosing not to disclose it. Hiding connotes fear or defensiveness motivated by unresolved personal conflicts, whereas nondisclosure implies a deliberate, conscious choice based on considerations of therapeutic benefit. She wrote of her feeling that, as a pregnant lesbian therapist, she was hiding something from her patients when she did not correct their assumptions that her pregnancy was proof of heterosexuality. "In my work with patients during my pregnancy I often felt I was not being emotionally honest or available to them. I felt constrained, as if I was hiding a part of myself from them. They had spoken of my personal life and made assumptions about it. . . . I was unsure of how much to disclose and how much to keep private" (p. 46).

Similarly, Gartrell (1984) pointed out that "wedding rings and office pictures of spouses and children are not invisible to clients" (p. 3) and that failure to be equally open about one's gay orientation is inevitably indicative of a double standard. Although references to spouses and children are no longer manifestly indicative of a heterosexual identity, in most people the default assumption is one of heterosexuality. Homosexuality, then, falls into the category of rarely considered possibilities, which, when unaddressed, reinforce the default, standard, dominant version of reality.

There exists also the danger that, when gay and lesbian therapists do not disclose their sexual orientation, patients may learn of it through external sources or social networks. If this occurs, then patients may assume that nondisclosure was caused by shame regarding the therapist's sexual orientation, thus making it far more difficult for this issue to be discussed in therapy and almost certainly affecting patients' ability to be open and honest about other sensitive topics.

Drescher (2002) discusses the personal benefits he derived from his experiences in therapy with both gay and straight therapists:

> My experience with my own two therapists sensitized me to how a patient's knowledge of the sexual orientation of a therapist can have an impact on treatment. In my first therapy, I needed someone I believed was like me [a gay man] to learn how to accept myself. In my analysis, on the other hand, the work with someone who I thought was not like me provided me a way of accepting otherness and differences, both in others and in myself. (p. 52)

As with many other intimate disclosures, a therapist's willingness to discuss his or her sexual identity creates opportunities for patients to more fully address a host of related issues, including sexuality, secret keeping, identity formation, and relationships with family members and friends.

Finally, it is important to note that contemporary discussions of sexual orientation can scarcely proceed without the specter of AIDS, HIV, and other sexually transmitted diseases. A therapist's disclosure of his or her gay identity may lead to patient questions regarding health status and ultimately greater patient disclosure about risk, health, and fears. Of course, requests for such information may or may not be met by therapist disclosures. As with other private, highly intimate, information (such as pregnancy), the decision whether and what to disclose regarding HIV status is ultimately a function of what therapists are comfortable with and what they believe the clinical consequences are of such disclosures.

Therapist Illness

Health and, even more fundamentally, life is the most basic requirement for the therapist to conduct therapy. As Friedman (1991) has noted: "The health and honesty of the therapist is a fundamental assumption that both parties bring to the therapeutic situation" (pp. 417–418). When health is compromised and life is threatened, the entire foundation of therapy is shaken. An ill therapist is inevitably more vulnerable, fragile, and needy than a healthy one; feeling vulnerable is universally uncomfortable, but it is a special challenge for a therapist attempting to project a strong, competent image for patients (Counselman & Alonso, 1993). Moreover, the facts of illness and neediness are inimical to those many individuals who enter the mental health field aware that they are better at meeting others' needs than they are at acknowledging their own. As is true of therapist pregnancy and sexual identity, there is a lack of clear therapeutic guidelines on what and when an ill therapist should tell his or her patients.

Nondisclosure of illness is a very seductive option. Like pregnant therapists, ill therapists may find it expedient to avoid disclosure and thereby avoid some of the intense emotional expressions—including compassion, sympathy, fear, and resentment—that would inevitably be directed toward them. They may feel so overburdened by illness that the idea of submitting to additional stresses (let alone facilitating them) becomes overwhelming. Furthermore, in cases of terminal illness, nondisclosure also allows the work to go on without painful discussions of termination and the need for the patient to find a new therapist. If by continuing to work one can convince oneself and one's patients that one is not really sick or really dying, then practicing therapy may become a way of "tricking" death. Friedman (1991), for example, wrote of her initial decision not to disclose her illness (cancer) to her patients, explaining it in terms of needing to concentrate all her energies on dealing with her illness and having none to spare for her patients' anticipated reactions, fears, and anxieties. She further reasoned that "knowledge of my illness would unnecessarily burden them" (p. 407), thus trying to reconcile her own personal needs and limited resources with the perceived benefits for her patients.

While somewhat compelling, Friedman's assumption that each of her patients would have the same reaction to her disclosure is questionable. Some would likely have felt burdened (as she noted), whereas others might well have used this information to explore painful, frightening feelings of their own and express previously unarticulated feelings toward their therapist. Moreover, while her decision may have been the best possible one in this case, it is nonetheless important to note the very natural tendency to rationalize the more expedient course of action as the "correct" one. Human mortality has long given rise to avoidance and denial; even in the face of fatal disease, few are able to truly comprehend and come to terms with the loss of their perceived "personal specialness." Therapists are as vulnerable to these illusions as are other mortals; many postpone, until it is too late, facing the finite nature of their existence. Some continue to see patients far past the point where they are truly able to help. Denial may have especially disastrous results if it leads to a therapist dying before any preparation of the patient has taken place.

The denial of mortality may also be one of the reasons for the relative dearth of published material on therapist illness and its impact on therapy. What is difficult to face is also difficult to write about, and therapists may be reluctant to do either. Indeed, even Freud himself, who was chronically ill for the last 17 years of his life (suffering from cancer of the jaw), never wrote about his illness and its influence on his therapeutic work (Counselman & Alonso, 1993; Halpert, 1982). This conspicuous silence may have served as a suggestion to future therapists that the appropriate course of action in this situation is to struggle on heroically, ignoring one's illness. By providing such a stoic "identificatory model," Freud may have provided a covert rationalization for avoidance, isolation, and denial among therapists who face serious illness.

Another easily imagined option for therapists: downplaying the severity of their illness via incomplete or sugarcoated disclosures. Despite a genuine intention to disclose realistically, a terminally ill therapist may end up imparting a false sense of optimism, stemming from an inability to avoid some degree of denial. This may lead to therapists colluding with their patients' fears of overwhelming the therapist, and subtly discouraging the expression of patient resentment, anger, and hostility. One example in the literature is of a therapist who disclosed his illness to his patients in what he believed was a clear and straightforward way. His patients, however, felt that their awareness of the nature of his illness (terminal metastatic cancer) and his prognosis was uncertain at best. They unanimously recalled that he did not use the word "cancer" to describe his tumor and that they felt encouraged to deny the severity of his illness by his optimistic attitude (Kaplan & Rothman, 1986). Therapists who convey inaccurate information about their serious medical condition help generate a state of "knowing, yet not really knowing" in their patients—arguably, the psychic state most antithetical to the goals of insight-oriented psychotherapy. Patients may deny the reality of a therapist's illness for many reasons, but one of them may be their (often correct) perception that full awareness will be intolerable to the therapist.

Of course, the difficult task of acknowledging mortality and preparing patients for separation (often before their therapeutic work is completed) must be faced not only by therapists who suffer from fatal diseases but also by relatively healthy therapists who are of advanced age. "Simply by aging, the psychoanalyst is slowly dying, and plans need to be made in advance" (Kaplan & Rothman, 1986, p. 561). That this simple truth has such startling power and is so eminently unpleasant to admit is further evidence of the ubiquitous desire to deny death (Becker, 1973). The problem is that, in doing so, one denies vital aspects of life as well. The idea that the denial of death is connected to a denial of life has been eloquently stated by the novelist Henry Miller (1941): "In the attempt to defeat death man has been inevitably obliged to defeat life, for the two are inextricably related. Life moves on to death, and to deny one is to deny the other" (p. 6).

That a therapist's illness may serve as a powerful stimulus for patients seems obvious. Clinical reports also suggest that ignoring or minimizing that stimulus may prove harmful to the patient's therapeutic progress (Halpert, 1982; Kaplan & Rothman, 1986). Because they are prone to intense identifications, patients with borderline pathology may be especially vulnerable to the consequences of unacknowledged therapist illness. Freud's famous patient, the Wolf Man, exhibited extreme hypochondria and somatic delusions following his referral by Freud to Ruth Mack Brunswick in 1926. Brunswick (1928) reports that the Wolf Man was shocked at Freud's appearance after the first operation on his mouth, and that a few months later this patient's own mouth and nose became focal somatic preoccupations. For the next 2 years, as Freud was undergoing surgical procedures for oral cancer, the Wolf Man (even when Freud was no longer his analyst) proceeded to visit doctors and dentists and had various operations performed on his mouth and nose. Neither Freud nor Brunswick (who had also been analyzed by Freud) made any direct references to the Wolf Man's overt identification with his former analyst's illness. It is difficult to imagine that this blatant avoidance of the subject was beneficial to the Wolf Man; indeed, Brunswick (1928) reports that his symptoms worsened and he appeared to be clinically regressing.

Full disclosure of a therapist's illness contains its own significant perils, including burdening patients with information they cannot process easily and inhibiting their discussion of problems that may appear insignificant compared with the therapist's life-threatening illness. Upon hearing the news of their therapist's illness, patients may feel guilty bringing up issues that are perceived as minor or relatively trivial, and may attempt to repress them or minimize their importance. This may in turn lead to feelings of resentment against the ill therapist, which could serve to further exacerbate feelings of guilt.

But therapist disclosure of illness may also greatly benefit both parties. It may provide a sort of gruesome service to those therapists who have become too caught up in the myth of their own invincibility. The forced encounter with their own weakness and mortality may contribute to a more human connection with patients. As the awareness of the limited time available for therapy becomes stronger, patience for "fluff" diminishes, even disappears completely; willingness to advise, interrupt and interpret, agree and disagree, be brutally honest, and become personally involved takes its place (Friedman, 1991; Halpert, 1982). The perception of death may result in a clarification of life and its priorities. Weinberg (1988) wrote about how the experience of an acute and chronic illness, including life-threatening episodes, influenced her outlook on life and her work with patients. In the final analysis, she felt that her experience provided her with certain "gifts" that ultimately made her a better therapist. She became "hypersensitive to patients' moods, reactions and transferential feelings," gained an "increased distance from cultural and societal dictates," and acquired a "more lucid focus on essential interpersonal issues" (p. 460). Most importantly, she noted, "this experience has sensitized me not only to illness and death, but to the importance of competence and self determination, and, most significantly, to life" (p. 460). Similarly, Friedman (1991) wrote that "I think I did some of my best therapeutic work that year [of my illness]; in the face of death, life takes on a special urgency and I was less likely to let things slip by" (p. 409). This is in direct contrast to the notion of an overburdened, weakened therapist struggling to deal with his or her illness and only too happy to let "unpleasant" things slip by.

A patient in a short story by therapist/writer Amy Bloom ("Psycho-analysis Changed My Life," 1993) is initially taken aback by the abrupt change in therapeutic style in her dying therapist—from silent, cautious, and calculating to very direct, even shockingly blunt. Ultimately, however, the patient becomes much improved as a result. Being forced by her dying therapist to move on, to stop wallowing in her old unproductive rumina-tions, and to actually live her life proves almost miraculous. It is as if the therapist, herself facing the impending loss of her life, cannot bear to see life wasted by her patient. In the end, her patient's blossoming is a "rebirth" that serves to ease the concerns of the dying therapist on her jour-ney toward death. Both patient and therapist benefit from the courage of the therapist's disclosure in this story.

The idea that a therapist's vulnerability and pain may sometimes be an advantage when working with sick patients has roots both in Eastern phi-losophies (where the concept of the "wounded healer" is widely accepted) and in classical mythology (Durban, Lazar, & Ofer, 1993). The Greek myth of the centaur Chiron illustrates well the "wounded healer" concept. After being mortally wounded in battle, Chiron was assigned the task of teaching mankind the art of medicine; his wound was seen as a source of wisdom to be imparted and shared with others. Having faced his mortality, he was in position to help others face theirs. It is often acknowledged that psychic wounds (when properly scarred) may strengthen or enrich therapists, but this ennobling quality is not usually attributed to bodily wounds. There is an artificiality to the distinction, as we recognize that physical and psycho-logical pain often coexist and interact in intricate ways.

In short, a seriously or terminally ill therapist with perspective, insight, awareness, and appropriate distance may enable patients to work though the most fundamental and terrifying problem of human life in the safest of settings. Patients of deceased therapists have reported that the therapist's disclosure of terminal illness and the facilitation of open discussion of all the attendant implications were helpful in dealing with such intense exis-tential issues as past losses, fears of abandonment and death, and the mean-ing of life. A therapist's disclosure of a life-threatening illness is also a poi-gnant reminder that complete emotional security is an unrealistic goal in life. Indeed, the acknowledgment and ultimate acceptance of suffering and death may sharpen and intensify the quality of a person's life. As Frieda Fromm-Reichmann (1952) wrote, "Acceptance of emotional insecurity, which is the acceptance of a certain amount of anxiety in the lives of the psychiatrist and his patients, is one of the constructive forces in the psychotherapeutic process" (p. 101).

Viktor Frankl (1997) noted that life need not be free of suffering to be meaningful; the same holds true for psychotherapy. Neither the inevitability of death nor the looming end of therapy dooms the therapeutic process; on the contrary, they may be seen as providing a profound, though perhaps profoundly painful, opportunity for growth. A terminally ill therapist who is willing and able to honestly explore the meanings and impact of death may be giving his or her patients the ultimate gift. As Tennyson (1842) wrote: "Death closes all: but something ere the end / Some work of noble note, may yet be done" (pp. 69–70).

CHAPTER 9

Supervisee and Supervisor Disclosure

The thought actually expressed was, so to speak, dragged into the front line by another thought that preferred not to reveal itself just yet.

—SARAMAGO (2002, p. 247)

We were no longer talking about anything. The language of discourse had shut out experience altogether.

—BELLOW (1982, p. 136)

Obscured by the attention paid to the issues of patient and therapist disclosure is the fact that therapist supervisors and supervisees must also consider what they will and will not reveal to each other. There is a considerable degree of isomorphism in the tensions that exist between each of these dyads: supervisees, like patients, are often guarded in their disclosures out of fear of shame and negative evaluation; supervisors, like therapists, struggle with how much to reveal. Furthermore, most supervisees, like most patients, are unlikely to reveal all their secrets—some feelings and thoughts will remain hidden, often obscured by a focus on less important, far safer, issues. And most supervisors, like most therapists, will presumably be more disclosing, personally giving, openly reassuring, and even humorous than the literature suggests or they have acknowledged to all but their closest friends or colleagues. Finally, in both situations, clinical work, or at least the quality of the dyadic relationship, is likely to suffer in the absence of a reasonable degree of disclosure.

SUPERVISEE DISCLOSURE

In Robertson Davies' (1972) book *The Manticore*, a Jungian therapist says to her patient: "If I am to help you, you will have to speak to me from your best self, honestly and with trust; if you continue to speak to me from your inferior, suspicious self . . . I shall not be able to do anything for you" (p. 19). The same remark might also be made by a supervisor to a supervisee. Nevertheless, all of us who have been supervised or otherwise evaluated in our jobs know that this admonition is both wise and simplistic. It contains an essential truth—learning is best accomplished when we are open and fully disclosing about what we do and don't know, about the mistakes we have made, about the ways we have thought about the tasks that need to be accomplished, about the feelings we bring to these tasks, and about what we believe we need to learn. But the sentence is also too glib. It overlooks aspects of shame inherent in all close relationships that interfere with the full expression of who we are and what we think and feel. It overlooks the fact that we all have felt and sometimes yielded to the sentiment that Tolstoy (1877), in *Anna Karenina*, expressed so well: "There were questions on which they could never meet and about which it was best not to talk" (p. 602). But it mostly overlooks the essential vulnerability supervisees feel while being supervised. In fact, "One could hypothesize that supervisees would leave even more things unsaid in supervision than clients do in therapy because of the evaluative consequences and involuntary nature of supervision" (Ladany, Hill, Corbett, & Nutt, 1996). Patients, after all, may leave therapies that feel unproductive or unsafe. Supervisees usually have no such option.

Still, it is true that in virtually every therapeutic model supervisors expect comprehensive and accurate information about therapy sessions and the trainee's internal processing of the case. Exposure of the psychotherapy trainee's work is the "sine qua non of good supervision" (Alonzo & Ruttan, 1988, p. 577). Or, in the words of Ladany et al. (1996): "Supervisors cannot help supervisees with concerns they do not know about" (p. 10). In some models, supervisors expect trainees to be forthright not only about their clinical work but also about their experience of the supervision itself. This expectation, one often held by psychodynamically oriented supervisors, is based on the belief that a supervisee will manifest many of the same interpersonal dynamics in the supervisory situation as he or she does in the clinical situation and that these need to be addressed as part of the supervisory process. The supervisee who acknowledges feeling insecure or shy or avoidant around the discussion of certain issues in supervision may become more aware that these issues are also manifest in his or her conduct of therapy.

Expectations aside, as in every other interpersonal situation, nondisclosure is normative and unavoidable in supervision. Some is due to the inherent difficulties in conveying to another the complexities of the therapeutic process and to the uncertainty about what should and shouldn't be reported (Wallace & Alonzo, 1994; Worthington, 1987; Yerushalmi, 1992). However, some nondisclosures are the result of conscious decisions to distort or withhold information, a product of the ubiquitous tension between secrecy and openness. Ladany et al. (1996) found that conscious omission by supervisees is nearly universal. They found that over 97% of a sample consisting primarily of doctoral students in counseling and clinical psychology reported withholding at least some information from their supervisors. According to Wallace and Alonso (1994), trainees will "more or less consciously omit discussion of significant information about their psychotherapy experiences to varying degrees, at different stages of training, with reference to certain psychotherapy patients and issues, and in relation to different supervisors" (p. 213). Thus, while some nondisclosure is inevitable, the timing and nature of the process may be affected by multiple personal and contextual variables.

Among the contributory factors underlying supervisee disclosure is that most inhibiting emotion—shame. Not surprisingly, it rears its head in the supervisory situation much as it does in a strictly therapeutic context. Learning to be a therapist necessarily involves exposing one's confusion, personal vulnerabilities, and professional ignorance to a usually highly experienced and well-regarded figure in the field. As Hahn (2001) has noted, the structure and format of supervision facilitates shame: "Supervisees experience a strong desire to be competent and autonomous along with fears of being found wanting in some respect" (p. 272). And, while this is true of virtually all professions as part of the apprenticeship process, there is a unique aspect of psychotherapeutic work that accentuates the potential shame: In psychotherapy one's very self is the essential tool in the work.

Although there are certainly technical skills to master, the work of the psychotherapist—the need to possess and demonstrate wisdom, empathy, tact, interpersonal sensitivity, strength, patience, flexibility, tolerance for ambiguity, and humor, among other qualities—draws so palpably upon an individual's skills as a caring, well-related human being. Thus, acknowledgment that one is struggling with the work all too often feels tantamount to admitting that one is struggling to be the human being one wants to be and should be. Expanding on this theme, Yourman and Farber (1996) suggested that some intense emotions experienced by trainees toward clients, including sexual or angry feelings, may be perceived by the trainee as nonprofessional or reflective of personal or professional inadequacy, and thus withheld from a supervisor's scrutiny. Consistent with these observations, Yourman (2003) found that supervisees with high shame scores disclose at significantly lower rates than supervisees who are less shame-prone.

What further exacerbates the potential for nondisclosure or distortion is the power that supervisors wield over supervisees. This power first resides in the immediacy of supervisory sessions in which a supervisor's comments can greatly affect the mood and self-esteem of a supervisee (sometimes for remarkably long periods of time). Ladany (2004), whose work on supervisor–supervisee disclosure has galvanized the field, revealed the following unfortunate supervisory experience (one, however, that fueled his desire to do research on this topic): "Supervision largely consisted of my supervisor beginning each sentence with 'What is it about you that is having difficulty with . . . ?' Occasionally, though, he would mix it up by attacking me personally" (p. 4). While some supervisees might be able to be openly disclosing under such circumstances, most would feel inhibited. We might even hypothesize that many would be quite tempted to distort experiences or only report successes.

A supervisor's power also resides in the evaluations that he or she provides to the training program (to be scrutinized by, among others, the trainee's advisee and the director of training) and, in the case of supervisees who are currently in doctoral programs in psychology, letters of recommendation that supervisees may be asked to send to internship sites. These letters can greatly affect a trainee's chances of being admitted to a preferred program. Rosenblatt and Mayer (1975) have observed that, because of their fear of negative evaluation and their realization that any information revealed to a supervisor could be used against them, trainees may be tempted to "engage in manipulative behavior" (p. 188).

While there are certainly "main effects" for how a supervisee approaches supervision, including his or her interpersonal style and psychological makeup (e.g., shame-proneness), and while the same is true for what a supervisor brings to this situation, there is also an interaction effect. That is, the extent to which a supervisee is open and honest to the supervisor is based not only on what each bring separately to the equation but also on the ways that the dyad works together. This is true, of course, for the therapist–patient dyad and for all other interpersonal situations. But in every training program there are almost always surprises in terms of effective supervisory matches—those that either exceed expectations regarding the effectiveness of the match or fail to fulfill expectations of a supposed ideal pairing.

Supervisee disclosure patterns, like those of patients, can take several problematic forms. There are supervisees who consistently omit significant clinical material and those on the other end of this spectrum who flood the supervisor with a plethora of details, feelings, insecurities, and questions. There are those who distort, exaggerate, or even fabricate experiences in the service of making themselves look better. And there are those supervisees—virtually all, according to Ladany et al. (1996)—who at least occasionally conceal their thoughts or reactions to the supervisor in the here and now of supervision. But whenever a trainee withholds or distorts material or feelings, there is the danger of a less than optimal learning experience for the trainee and, in a worse case scenario, compromised treatment of patients (Yourman & Farber, 1996).

All these considerations lead to an exquisite tension in the supervisory process between students' desire to be open (and, in so doing, improve their clinical skills and validate their courage and willingness to grow) and their often equally strong desire to appear competent to themselves and their supervisor (and, in so doing, increase the likelihood of their receiving positive evaluations, a favorite internship, and a good job).

Assumedly, most supervisors are aware of these tensions. But they, too, must negotiate some difficult balancing acts. They must be accepting as well as appropriately critical (i.e., point out clinical errors). Similarly, they must push the supervisee hard enough for him or her to learn new ways of thinking and behaving but not push so hard that resistances and resentment set in. They must make the supervisee's mistakes seem normative but not reduce him or her to a stereotype (e.g., "All beginners tend to do that"). They must sometimes allow the new therapist a degree of creativity and flexibility while not being indiscriminately approving of all interventions based on good intent.

In addition, supervisors must find an appropriate balance between focusing on a supervisee's personal issues and therapeutic skills, an extremely difficult task. As Greben and Ruskin (1994) have noted, personal issues of trainees that require extensive supervisory attention are probably best left to the purview of individual therapy. Overall, though, supervisors know that too much personal confrontation or focus may lead to undue anxiety and secrecy, whereas "a supervision that is virtually conflict-free may be indicative that difficult issues are being eschewed to avoid anxiety" (Yourman & Farber, 1996, p. 569).

Jean Seibel, a supervisor whom I interviewed, approaches these tasks in the following ways:

> "My job is to create an atmosphere of emotional safety, a relaxed environment where the student is not put on the spot. I tell my supervisees: 'It's my responsibility to guide you; there's a process in learning how to use supervision and I will guide you.' I ask them their expectations, what they'd like from supervision. I tell them that if there's something that hasn't been addressed they should let me know . . . they know there's an evaluative component—we go over the nature of the evaluation measure. I tell them there shouldn't be any surprises—it's a process we're engaged in from the time we begin our work together. In the beginning, in particular, I'm always asking whether they have any questions for me . . . One of the things I've done that most helps with their willingness to disclose to me is that I'm clear about the boundary between supervision and therapy. In most supervisions, I've had the opportunity to say 'This piece of what you're talking about is for supervision, and this piece is for your own therapy.' This invariably

makes them freer to bring something up because it creates more safety. They don't have to worry about whether they should or shouldn't bring something up. They know they won't be chastised or criticized for bringing up 'inappropriate' material. And they know that I'll try my hardest to keep them from spilling their personal stuff in supervision, sometimes protecting them from their own need to look as honest as possible . . . The most important piece of supervision, though—the one that allows students to continue to be disclosing and honest—is refraining from criticism. Not criticizing is critical. Even more important than complimenting them. You can always add a well-deserved compliment. It's much harder, in fact impossible, to take back a criticism."

SUPERVISEE DISCLOSURE: WHAT THE RESEARCH SAYS

As noted above, Ladany et al. (1996) found that virtually their entire sample acknowledged withholding some type of information from their supervisors. These nondisclosures were most often related to negative reactions to supervisors (e.g., "He is very rigid and narrow in theory and practice") and personal issues (e.g., "I'm pregnant"). Other withheld information pertained to evaluation concerns (e.g., "I wonder how my supervisor will evaluate me"), clinical mistakes (e.g., "I sometimes feel I made a mistake in a session, but rather than discuss it in supervision I wait until the next therapy session to try to correct it"), and general client observations (e.g., "The extent of sexual activity my clients discuss").

Analogous to Hill et al.'s (1993) findings regarding the difficulties patients have in expressing their negative feelings to their therapists, Ladany et al. (1996) reported that the material most frequently not disclosed in supervision was trainees' negative reactions to supervisors. Fully 90% of their sample reported this phenomenon. They also noted that supervisees believed they were more likely to withhold negative reactions to supervisors they perceived as less attractive, less interpersonally sensitive, and less task-oriented. These authors further indicated that this particular form of nondisclosure was likely to occur as a result of "deference" to the supervisor, impression management, and "fear of political suicide" (i.e., protecting one's career). Furthermore, supervisees whose nondisclosures tended to be of this type were less satisfied with supervision.

Relatedly, Moskowitz and Rupert (1983) found that when supervisory conflicts were not discussed the consequences were significant: 33.3% of trainees in such situations acknowledged censoring reports and/or process notes, and 25% reported a pattern of spurious compliance with their supervisor. Taken together, these findings suggest that face-to-face acknowledgment of negative feelings—whether in the therapeutic or supervisory dyad—is not only extremely difficult for most individuals but when avoided increases the likelihood of subsequent disingenuous interactions.

In general, participants in Ladany et al.'s research attributed nondisclosures to their sense that these topics were unimportant, too personal, involved feelings that were too negative, or that the supervisory alliance was not sufficiently strong to contain these thoughts. Again, the pattern of responses here is remarkably consistent to that of patients in psychotherapy. Individuals in both these settings avoid raising issues that feel too intimate and potentially upsetting, and issues that feel threatening to the integrity of the dyad. Not surprisingly, supervisors in Ladany et al.'s study who were perceived as more open and collaborative elicited less nondisclosure.

Yourman and Farber's (1996) research investigated two primary questions: To what extent does supervisee nondisclosure occur? What factors are predictive of nondisclosure? Their sample ($n = 93$), most of whom were in doctoral programs in clinical and counseling psychology, completed a questionnaire in reference to a specific supervisor with whom they were working at that time. Results indicate that most of the time supervisees communicate to their supervisors what they believe to be an honest picture of their clinical and supervisory experiences. For example, on a 1–7 scale (1 = never; 4 = sometimes; 7 = always) respondents in this study had a mean score of 5.3 on the item "I am comfortable discussing my feelings of inadequacy as a clinician." On another item, "When I have interacted with clients in ways I thought my supervisor might disapprove of, I have been honest in describing these interactions," the mean score was also high (5.1).

However, results of this study also confirm Ladany et al.'s (1996) finding that it is far from rare for a supervisee to withhold clinical material from a supervisor. Perhaps the item in the Yourman and Farber study that is most indicative of a supervisee's tendency toward nondisclosure is "I have omitted describing details of my work that I have felt were clinical errors." Whereas 60% of the sample never or only infrequently failed to inform supervisors of perceived clinical errors, the remaining 40% reported that they withheld this information at a moderate to high frequency. In addition, over 47% of this sample reported telling their supervisor what he or she wanted to hear at a moderate to high frequency. Moreover, 59% of the sample reported that they never or only infrequently felt comfortable disclosing negative feelings toward their supervisor. Thus, in supervisory situations that may have especially high potential for shame and conflict, as many as 30–40% of supervisees withhold information at a moderate to high level, and as many 50% are at a moderate to high level in terms of telling their supervisor what he or she seems to want to hear.

At first glance, Ladany et al.'s (1996) finding that 97% of supervisees withhold information seems high. However, in Yourman and Farber's (1996) study over 91% reported that they do not always inform their supervisor when they have interacted with patients in ways they believe the supervisor will disapprove. Consistent, too, with Ladany et al.'s data, Yourman and Farber found that the material most frequently withheld was related to events in supervision and the supervisory relationship.

Yourman and Farber suggested that supervisors might address the shame-based aspects of supervision by speaking directly to their supervisees about the issues of disclosure and evaluation. They also suggested that supervisors attempt "to maintain or restore, when necessary, supervisees' positive feelings toward their own therapeutic competence, and positive feelings between supervisor and supervisee" (p. 573). For example, when a supervisee reports a clinical error, the supervisor should help him or her view such mistakes as inevitable and as opportunities for learning. Geller's (2005a) way of socializing new patients by explaining some of the roles and expectations involved in being in therapy also has much to offer as a paradigm for supervisors to use with their supervisees. As he explains: "To prepare 'naïve' patients for the exploratory work to come, I will try to underscore the courage it takes to speak truthfully about one's 'vulnerable selves.' Also, I will emphasize the inevitability of reluctances about speaking 'truthfully' given the degree of candor and affective freedom required of patients. I will typically find an occasion to mention that so-called resistances and 'negative transference reactions' are inevitable, and that they may bring to light otherwise inaccessible knowledge (pp. 387–388)." Preparing trainees for the work of supervision as well as periodically reviewing this work ("How are we doing?" "Are there experiences that you're struggling to find a way to talk about in here?") are both means of increasing the likelihood of honest interchanges and effective and gratifying supervision.

One might expect that video- or audiotaping sessions would minimize supervisee nondisclosure or distortion. However, Yourman and Farber (1996) found that taping is not significantly related to supervisee nondisclosure (nor satisfaction with supervision). This is not entirely surprising when one considers that supervisors cannot listen to every moment of a tape, that the inner feelings of supervisees are not captured by tape, and that taping itself may be perceived as an intrusion and actually contribute to a climate of apprehension and mistrust.

The authors of this study found that no demographic variable was significantly related to disclosure in supervisees. The variables analyzed included supervisee age, gender, ethnicity, and number of years in a training program; supervisor gender; supervisor–supervisee gender interactions; and matching versus mismatching of theoretical orientation. What did prove to be significant was supervisee satisfaction with supervision—the greater the extent of satisfaction, the greater the extent of perceived disclosure. This result confirms the findings of Ladany et al. (1996) and Moskowitz and Rupert (1983) in demonstrating that a strong supervisory alliance is significantly related to trainee disclosure. This result is also, of course, parallel to that found in studies of patient disclosure (e.g., Farber & Hall, 2002). Another variable that shows preliminary evidence of being linked to disclosure is supervisees' sexual attraction toward their supervisors. Ladany (2004) found that supervisees are typically sexually attracted to the physical and interpersonal characteristics (e.g., genuineness, sense of humor) of their supervisors and that this attraction leads to a stronger alliance and increased self-disclosure.

A SUPERVISOR'S PERSPECTIVE

Some of the issues noted above, especially those related to the importance of the supervisory alliance, are illustrated in this example. However, here ethnicity did seem to affect the alliance and subsequent supervisee disclosure. Perhaps though it would be more accurate to hypothesize that it was the absence of discussions about ethnicity and ethnic differences in the earliest stages of this relationship that damaged the working alliance and hindered disclosure.

In this case, one brought to my attention by a colleague, a white supervisor was working with a black supervisee in a facility where the professional staff was almost entirely white. She (the supervisor) began to be aware that her supervisee was acting "very closed" in supervision. More specifically, the supervisor noticed that she exhibited flat affect, that her responses to questions seemed calculated, and that they contained little emotional or factual content. In addition, she noted that there were many silences in their work together. The supervisor, sensing that their stuckness might be racially influenced, asked her supervisee: "How do you feel about the fact that you're black, I'm white, and I'm supervising you?" This intervention proved initially effective: "It poured out that that was the key to her reticence. We talked about the racial issue. She acknowledged that it bothered her. She felt that I couldn't understand her experience."

During this discussion, the supervisee related a specific incident that occurred on the inpatient ward in which they both worked. The supervisee thought that the supervisor was going to get physically hurt by a client but was told by the supervisor not to intervene even if there was a physical situation. The supervisee acknowledged feeling "patronized" by this mandate. In turn, the supervisor was "surprised" and "shocked" at the supervisee's reaction: She (the supervisor) thought she was being responsible for and protective of her trainee. "My perception of being helpful was perceived as diminishing her in her eyes." During the 6 months following their discussion, the relationship did get better, but according to the supervisor her trainee was never entirely amenable to her help or suggestions and was not entirely forthcoming either about her clinical cases or their relationship.

A SUPERVISEE'S PERSPECTIVE

The following observations on disclosure in psychotherapy supervision were written by a first-year doctoral student in clinical psychology. They are based on her reactions to her first supervisory experiences.

On disclosure and trust: "I really believe in the importance of sharing my truest feelings and fears with my supervisor, because how else will I truly learn? I would say that this kind of pull toward interpersonal honesty has always been for me a kind of default position. But in the supervisory relationship, I find that what opposes this instinct in me is a voice that asks, 'Can I trust this person?' Can I trust him or her not only as I would my own therapist, but as someone who is 'on my side' professionally? Will he or she mistake my insecurities for irreconcilable faults, judge me 'unfit' for this work in some way, or, scariest of all, write an evaluation of me that either explicitly or implicitly, overtly or subtly, conveys these impressions? Because supervision involves the ever-present backdrop of 'evaluation' in addition to the discussion of personal issues, the level of trust I feel I need to have in a supervisor almost seems to exceed that which I would need to have in my own therapist. More succinctly put, supervision feels to require personal *and* professional trust.

On disclosing thoughts in the here and now: "One of my supervisors occasionally directs questions to me about my reactions to her in the moment. One such question followed a period of about three weeks during which she had either been (negligibly) late for appointments with me or, on one occasion, visibly tired from having been up all night with her child who was sick (as she had explained to me in that session). At our next meeting, she acknowledged these occurrences and asked me how I was feeling about them—whether I was experiencing her as unavailable, etc. This was early on in our relationship, and I remember feeling a bit taken aback at her forthrightness. Until that point, I hadn't consciously given the incidents much thought, so I answered as honestly as I could in the moment that I hadn't been bothered. It was striking to me that she had brought this up, because I didn't anticipate being engaged by a supervisor in that way. But I was happy to have the sense that she was truly concerned about my feelings and interested in building a strong alliance, and it also gave me some insight into the nature of her analytical style. One other thought that struck me about this incident was the question of whether I could have been as honest in my answer as I was had my true feelings been less neutral. I think, occurring as this incident did early on in the relationship and taking me by surprise, that out of caution and awareness that I could not yet anticipate the ramifications, I would not have fully expressed my negative sentiments."

On disclosure and process: "A pivotal disclosure I remember making early on to my supervisor was about my experience of supervision itself. I said that I had been feeling unsure as to what 'supervision' really *meant*. What were the parameters, what were the goals, what kind of material was I expected to bring or would I most benefit from? I (sort of) knew the answers to these questions 'in theory,' or 'in general,' but because I was now faced with a specific situation—a unique person with whom I was forming a unique relationship—I felt it necessary to evaluate these questions with respect to 'us.' My disclosure was very well-received, and we had a fruitful discussion that has really helped me in the sessions that have followed. But what was also interesting about this incident was that, after that session, I perceived a change in the way my supervisor regarded me. It seemed as though my having brought up this issue (and also, I think, having talked about it as frankly as I did) engendered in her a heightened level of respect for me, a sense that I was taking the work seriously. I sensed that she now felt that we were like-minded, or that we could discuss things on a 'higher plane,' and I noticed that the feeling of our relationship had palpably changed from one of relative distance to one of greater closeness.

"The way my disclosure was received by her gave me a feeling of confidence that was, and continues to be, extremely valuable to me as a therapist-in-training. I feel that having gained her respect, I can be more honest and open in supervision. I feel that whatever I say will be viewed against the backdrop of that respect, which makes me less afraid to reveal my insecurities, my self-doubts—the negative things I perceive about myself and my work. And I think being able to discuss these things in particular is how I will ultimately be able to become a better therapist."

SUPERVISOR DISCLOSURE

Supervisors have the same essential task as others members in the psychotherapeutic system—to determine, within a complex and intense interpersonal context, what they will and will not disclose to their dyadic partner. Supervisors are in a more frankly educational role than are therapists, a situation that, depending on the individual's predilection, could either serve to facilitate or inhibit disclosure. Arguably, most supervisors view a large part of their role as modeling clinical skills through sharing their own experiences. Some, however, may be more didactic than interpersonally open, and still others may assume a traditional psychoanalytic stance that eschews open dialogue and disclosure.

Among other reasons, supervisors disclose to forge closer bonds with their supervisees; share professional wisdom; model therapeutic skills; and provide feedback to supervisees on their clinical work, interpersonal style, and psychological assets and blind spots. In doing so, they may feel wise, helpful, genuine, and intimate. They also are likely to feel that they are fulfilling an important professional responsibility. Still, research has shown that some types of disclosures are relatively easy to make (e.g., feedback about clinical problems), whereas other disclosures (e.g., professional concerns about the supervisee) are quite difficult. Indeed, supervisors have acknowledged that they are prone to withholding this latter type of information. In addition, supervisors are more likely to be open in their evaluations of trainee competence and progress to the extent that trainees are seen as being able to take in both positive and critical feedback with a minimal degree of defensiveness (Hoffman, Hill, Holmes, & Freitas, 2005).

This iterative process of supervisor openness and supervisee nondefensiveness may also be influenced by several nonobvious factors. For example, it may be difficult for a supervisee to simply accept a supervisor's suggestions or criticisms if he or she has received different or perhaps exclusively positive feedback from other supervisors. It may also be difficult for some supervisees to accept criticism from someone younger or someone with a different professional background (e.g., social work). Similarly, it may be difficult for trainees to accept feedback from a supervisor who espouses a very different theoretical perspective. What is often necessary to ensure mutual openness in these types of situations is for the participants to begin supervision by discussing their personal or theoretical differences and affirming a mutual willingness to respect and learn from each other's perspective. In this sense, the work involved here—the need to discuss early on in the relationship those demographic, stylistic, or theoretical differences that may interfere with the tasks at hand—is no different from that involved in the therapeutic dyad.

It is also true that, as in other interpersonal contexts, a strong relationship facilitates disclosure, while shame constricts it. As Hahn (2001) has noted, shame is not confined to the supervisee within the supervisory dyad. Supervisors often struggle to identify and acknowledge their own shame and may even allow their supervisees to shoulder a disproportionate amount of this emotion. That is, whatever shame may have been cocreated or coexperienced by the supervisory dyad may be placed exclusively upon the supervisee's shoulders to understand and work through. In many ways, this situation parallels that which occurs when therapists and patients

become aware of therapeutic impasses. Typically—or at least historically—this event would prompt therapists to examine the nature and extent
of the patient's resistance, assiduously avoiding an analysis or discussion of
their own role in this occurrence.

Supervisors are likely to feel shame when they feel inadequate in their
connection to their trainees or in any of their overlapping roles as teacher,
mentor, and evaluator (Alonzo & Ruttan, 1988). Most care deeply about
their work, are accomplished and highly regarded professionally, and
expect the work of supervision to be arduous but successful and rewarding.
When these expectations are not fulfilled, contemporary supervisors, more
than their counterparts from generations past, are likely to consider their
part in the process. Most have been immersed in a professional culture that
has emphasized collaborative relationships and the role of both participants in creating such structures. Moreover, supervisors—at least those
who are hired from outside a particular training setting—often get paid little or nothing for their efforts. They serve in this role for a variety of reasons, including a desire to be part of a university or medical setting (and
perhaps receive some benefits such as library or gym privileges), a need to
break the often lonely routine of private practice, a genuine wish to pass on
what they have learned to a new generation, and, as noted above, the pleasure of feeling helpful. Thus, for the most part, the rewards of supervision
are based not on remuneration but on the satisfaction of work well done.
Expectations may therefore be especially high, and thus the potential for
disappointment and shame.

Supervisors who experience anxiety or concerns related to their own
self-efficacy may not offer potentially useful feedback or personal observations to trainees (Ladany & Melincoff, 1999). They may become constricted and apprehensive in regard to their disclosures. Of course, the
most salient question here is whether supervisory disclosure is important
in any real clinical sense. Compared to those of patients, therapists, and
even supervisees, the disclosures of supervisors seem to be of minor import, with far less direct impact on the ultimate reference point: patient
welfare. "The link between supervision process and outcome on the one
hand and psychotherapy process and outcome on the other is tenuous"
(Ladany, 2004, p. 14). Nevertheless, even if supervisor disclosures have,
at best, only mild to moderate effects on supervision or therapy outcomes, well-timed supervisor disclosures can exert a powerful influence
on supervisees, affecting their own disclosures, the supervisory alliance,
and their professional development (Ladany & Walker, 2003). In this
sense, these disclosures can be seen as contributing to a chain of events
that, ideally, culminates in effective clinical care and effective professional
training. In fact, some evidence exists for one part of this link: When supervisors disclose more frequently, trainees experience a more effective
supervisory working alliance (Ladany & Lehrman-Waterman, 1999).

They perceive a greater agreement on the goals and tasks of supervision and a stronger emotional bond.

Supervisors do disclose. In Ladany and Lehrman-Waterman's (1999) study, 91% of their sample of trainees reported at least one instance of supervisory disclosure. The most frequent disclosure—reported by 73% of these respondents—involved personal issues of the supervisor (e.g., a supervisor's divorce, number of children, or vacation destination). The authors of this study, while noting that this type of disclosure is common, also questioned its value on several grounds: that it takes time away from more relevant supervisory issues; that, on the face of it, it seems to meet the supervisor's needs more than the supervisee's; and that, in some cases at least, it places a burden on the supervisee to care for the supervisor. Thus, the arguments here mirror earlier proscriptions leveled against therapist disclosures—namely, that they have too great a potential for gratifying the therapist's needs while derailing the essential purpose of the session.

The second most commonly reported supervisor disclosure (by 55% of respondents) was what the authors termed "neutral counseling experiences." Included in this category were comments about the supervisor's own experiences as a therapist, such as how he or she worked with a depressed or suicidal client or dealt with a client's persistent lateness to sessions. Ladany and Lehrman-Waterman viewed these disclosures far more favorably because they can be seen as a form of modeling, providing the trainee with new schema for dealing with common clinical situations. Again, these disclosures can be regarded as analogous to therapist disclosures that provide patients with new ways of understanding or negotiating frustrating situations.

Slightly more than half the respondents in this study (51%) reported that their supervisors had shared experiences relating to their own struggles with clients—an even more useful variant of the category ("neutral counseling experiences") described above. Supervisors who acknowledge their own difficulties with clients not only provide new models for dealing with tough situations but also allow supervisees to know, firsthand, how normative it is to feel vulnerable and fallible in working with clients. These disclosures, then, may lessen unrealistic expectations about clinical work and even about the supervisor's expertise. The authors do caution, however, that at times such disclosures can backfire, causing supervisees to become more anxious by the awareness that their supervisors may not have all the requisite answers.

Another category of supervisor disclosure is what these authors deem "counseling successes" (reported by 25% of respondents in their sample). These are comments (e.g., "I've been successful with depressed clients by being consistently empathic"; "I don't get in a test of wills with borderline patients and work with them quite well") that are on the border between acknowledging that one has done good work and evidencing a bit too much conceit in the reporting. Thus, disclosures in this category promote the view of supervisor as expert, a decidedly mixed blessing. At their best, these remarks allow supervisees to model expert work and even the confidence of the speaker; at their worst, they reflect a dubious tradition of therapists' assuming a mantle of omniscience, one that might cause quite competent supervisees to distance themselves from such supervisors.

More rarely, supervisors disclose on matters related to the supervisory relationship (12% of the sample) and their own experiences as a supervisor (8%). As the authors point out, the first category is akin to therapist's self-involving disclosures, a valuable source of information to many patients. Here, they note that direct discussion of the supervisory relationship (e.g., "I'm sorry that I wasn't more supportive of you the other day") may provide a means for repairing a rupture in this alliance. It may also provide a helpful model for the discussion of interpersonal "process," often a very difficult topic for novice therapists to undertake with their own clients. The latter category—supervisors' accounts of supervising (e.g., "I've been told by previous supervisees that I don't offer enough hands-on advice")—is one that the authors are more disparaging toward. Although they concede that it might lead to useful discussions with supervisees about the nature of supervision, they mostly regard it as a means for the supervisor to either distance him- or herself from the work or feel narcissistically gratified through self-focus.

The results of this study also indicated that supervisors who are supportive and warm tend to disclose more frequently and that those who share their own clinical struggles generate a strong emotional bond with their supervisees. While the authors strongly advocate the use of supervisor disclosures, viewing it as a means for establishing and maintaining a good alliance, they also realize that far more work needs to be done in this area. Research has not yet established what or when such disclosures are most effective nor whether there is a ceiling effect for their frequency or intensity. For the most part, the same could be said about patient, therapist, and supervisee disclosures—although work in these other areas far outpaces work in the area of supervisor disclosure.

Research has also investigated supervisor nondisclosures. Ladany and Melincoff (1999) found that the most common self-reported nondisclosures were supervisors' negative evaluations of trainees' clinical and overall professional work (74% of supervisors surveyed), supervisor personal issues (67%), and negative reactions to trainees' supervision performance (56%). Whereas the second category makes intuitive sense—supervisors should usually refrain from disclosing personal information to supervisees—the other two aspects of nondisclosure seem to suggest a failure in fulfilling a basic task of supervision, that of pointing out to students their errors, misjudgments, knowledge gaps, and beginners' mistakes. While keeping in mind that these nondisclosures may have occurred only occasionally, they are still problematic. Positive feedback and affirmations are powerful interpersonal reinforcers and deserve an honored place in a supervisor's repertoire, but they cannot serve in lieu of critical (i.e., negative) feedback to supervisees. Indeed, one could argue that the failure to offer negative perceptions of a supervisee's performance not only reflects poorly on the supervisor but also shows a fundamental disrespect for a supervisee's ability to hear and profit from this information.

Aggregated over all types of supervisor nondisclosures, the most common attribution for these events included supervisors' perceptions that they were not relevant (77%), that they were the supervisor's own issues (71%), and that they would elicit negative trainee reactions (64%). The first two reasons are quite understandable. However, the third reason offered for nondisclosure (negative trainee reaction) poses problems similar to those noted in the preceding paragraph. Whereas this could be seen as a manifestation of good supervisory judgment ("she's not ready to hear this"; "she'll discover this information when she's 'developmentally ready' "), it could also be seen as a reflection of insecurity or lack of integrity ("I'm not willing to bear the fallout of her hearing this"). To reiterate the point made earlier, supervisors who avoid providing such feedback risk patronizing students and, worse, risk robbing them of learning opportunities. But, as was true in the case of patients, therapists, and supervisees, here again lies probable evidence of just how difficult it is to offer face-to-face feedback that contains elements of negative evaluation.

In interviewing several supervisors for this chapter, several themes emerged consistently. Perhaps the most common theme—other than that supervision was almost always seen as a professionally fulfilling activity—was mild to moderate regret over not pushing students a bit harder, that is, not providing enough critical feedback. Most supervisors were aware that, at least occasionally, they held back comments, especially from their more talented students. "Things were going so well and she was such a talented student; I realized later that I had gotten into too comfortable a rhythm of listening, complimenting, occasionally making suggestions or asking questions."

Another theme that was frequently articulated by this group of psychodynamically oriented supervisors was that they were conflicted at times between wanting to share their own stories of clinical successes and their apprehension that doing so too often might make them seem arrogant or even patronizing. One supervisor said, "There are times that even as I'm talking I hear my father's voice saying 'When I was your age . . . ,' and I don't like that feeling." In response to a question about personal disclosures, many supervisors said that they often do share some of the small details of their lives, especially in the early sessions as they are asking questions about the supervisee. It is a way, they noted, of the two participants getting to know each other. According to many supervisors, this kind of information (e.g., "where I got my degree"; "a bit about my career path";

"books I've read recently") often continues to be a small but contextually important aspect of the relationship. More personal issues (e.g., information about children; professional gossip) are considered off-limits by almost all supervisors.

Many supervisors I spoke with thought that two particular types of disclosures were most effective: those that spoke to the supervisor's own experiences of clinical work; and those that took the form of emotionally resonant, empathic disclosures. In this second category are statements like "yes, the work is so very hard, so emotionally draining"; "I know, progress is so elusive sometimes; "that kind of thing frustrates me too." Supervisors felt a great sense of accomplishment when they shared a clinical experience that "worked" for their supervisee. But they also felt gratified when a suggestion of theirs didn't work but led to mutual processing about what happened and what next steps might be taken. Some of these themes are captured in the following example.

A CLINICAL EXAMPLE

A supervisor for the clinical psychology program I work for (Teachers College, Columbia University) offered the following example. The supervisor, a white male in his mid-40s, was working with a white female second-year graduate student in her late 20s:

"I chose this supervision to discuss because it was a particularly difficult one for me. It was clear that the student was extremely bright—very well read and with a wealth of research experience. It was also clear that the student enjoyed her clinical work. But it was clear, too, that the student had very little insight into her clinical limitations; in fact, she consistently overestimated her acumen and the extent to which her patients were benefiting from the therapy. There was a substantial discrepancy between her sense of her clinical abilities and my sense of this. Moreover—and here was where the hardest problem lay—she was often quite defensive in the face of suggestions or even slight negative feedback. My sense was that she was emotionally fragile. Whatever suggestions I made—gently I thought and interspersed with genuine approval of her commitment and caring—were met with a variant of 'I've already tried that' or 'I've already thought of that and I don't think it will work.' I tried—again I thought gently—to point out this pattern to her, letting her know that I thought she wasn't really taking in what I was offering and that I felt devalued. She claimed that this hadn't occurred in other supervisions, a claim I subsequently was to learn just wasn't true. I tried the following: I acknowledged that I struggled considerably as a young graduate student to allow myself to feel vulnerable in supervision. I wondered out loud whether she too experienced this. 'Yes, a bit, but I feel it hasn't gotten in the way of my learning.' This was just a case, she thought, that she felt particularly on top of and perhaps didn't need that much help with. I felt intensely ambivalent about what to do. I decided though that to let this pattern ride was to collude with her resistance. I said to her that while I commended her on her confidence, I also wondered whether there were any other feelings behind her self-assured demeanor. She began crying. Unfortunately, though, it soon became clear that the tears were meant not to signal that I had touched something important, if well-hidden, but rather that I had hurt her with these insinuations and that I should back off.

"I did back off then but at the next session I asked how she experienced what had happened. She was a 'little hurt' but understood that these 'miscommunications sometimes happen between people' and that it was 'OK.' It was beginning to feel like therapy to me and I wasn't sure that I wanted to keep going that way. I told her as much—told her that I did think she had some issues about appearing wrong or incompetent or vulnerable that probably should be addressed in her own therapy. She said something to the effect that she'd take this advice 'under advisement.' The balance of the semester was spent mostly in neutral. She would explain or show me (via videotape) her work, I would say things like, 'Hmm-hmm, that was good but I think I would have also have . . .' or, 'If you said that to me, I think I'd feel a bit hurt.' She was consistently noncommittal about my suggestions. And I didn't push any further. In retrospect, I don't think I was particularly helpful. Perhaps what I did best was to keep letting her know what I thought about her work despite her fighting me. Perhaps at some point, especially if another supervisor gives her the same sort of feedback, she may begin to take some of it in."

We see in this example, and the others in this chapter as well, so many of the issues that came up in the context of patient and therapist disclosures. Especially evident is the tension between candor and vulnerability, a tension that plays out so very differently among individuals. While it is easy to imagine that most supervisors and supervisees move toward the more candid end of the continuum as they gain experience and confidence in their respective roles, it is also entirely possible that some remain where they began, either stuck out of fear or comfortable with the degree of disclosure they've established for themselves.

CHAPTER 10

Conclusions

None of us can ever express the exact measure of his needs or his
thoughts or his sorrows; and human speech is like a cracked
kettle on which we tap crude rhythms for bears to dance to,
while we long to make music that will melt the stars.
—FLAUBERT (1856, p. 242)

There will always come a moment when we must ask ourselves if
the dream, the ambition, the secret hope of all secrets is, in fact,
the possibility, however vague, however remote, of ceasing to be a
secret.
—SARAMAGO (2002, p. 282)

The basic issue addressed in this book is disclosure in psychotherapy. What
do patients and therapists reveal to each other? What do supervisors and
supervisees reveal to each other? Upon what factors do they base their decisions? What are the consequences of their disclosures and nondisclosures?
Underlying these specific questions is the idea that disclosure is essential to
human relationships, a fundamental building block of identity and con-
nectedness and a frequent means of alleviating personal stress. What has
emerged in these chapters is that even in the context of that most confidential of setting, a therapist's office, difficult choices are constantly being
made and difficult emotions constantly faced. Patients, therapists, supervisors, and supervisees are all ostensibly committed to truth and openness in
their relationships with one another, and yet most struggle mightily—on a
conscious and unconscious level—with a fundamental human question:
What am I willing to let another know about me?

As has been documented throughout this book, there are numerous
factors that affect the answer to this question. If for the moment, though,
we observe from a broad macroanalytic level, we can identify two strong

countervailing cultural forces that influence individuals' disclosure patterns. On the one hand, there is a push for total emotional honesty, an ideal promulgated by Freud over 100 years ago, nourished by successive generations of psychodynamic clinicians, carried to some extremes by a 60s generation that developed encounter groups and celebrated the virtues of unbridled honesty, and still seen today in cultural phenomena ranging from instant messaging to reality television to online diaries (blogging). On the other hand, a strong backlash to "tell-all intimacy" has emerged, one that begs for limits to public confessions, is skeptical of the assumed benefits of disclosure, and sees repression and even denial as far more adaptive than Freud ever imagined. Patients may be more torn between these two positions more than therapists, supervisors, or supervisees if only because the latter group is immersed in a psychotherapeutic subculture that has historically privileged the first position. Still, it is hard for anyone to be entirely unaffected by strong cultural influences. Thus, whereas therapists, supervisors, and supervisees are likely to tout the advantages of disclosure for patients, they may also be more respectful of nondisclosure than their predecessors and very likely to believe that their own professional roles necessitate far less than total disclosure. Ultimately, then, all players in the psychotherapeutic matrix are subject to strong, often opposing, cultural dictates.

Culture, of course, is not the only influence on disclosure. Individual personality factors play a major role in this process, as do role expectations. Strong roles (that of therapist, patient, supervisor, and supervisee) may place strong constraints on disclosure. The constraints are necessarily different in each case: Patients are required to be self-disclosing, but here the requirement itself may pose the constraint—the expectation for full disclosure may feel too burdensome, too pressured, or too shameful. In the case of the therapist, although old rigid prohibitions against disclosure are thankfully changing, some vestiges of this tradition tend to endure, both within the psychoanalytic and CBT communities. In addition, the contemporary managed-care focus on short-term therapy and symptom reduction often leaves less room for therapist disclosure and mutual discussion of the therapeutic interaction. Many supervisors struggle to balance their need to listen with their desire to share their own experiences. Their dilemma may be confounded with the "rules" they have learned about the proper degree of disclosure allowed a therapist. And supervisees, like patients, face a role conflict that pits their desire to learn through disclosing against their fear of negative evaluation, self-consciousness, and shame.

Cultural and role-mediated influences on psychotherapy disclosure represent but two of its many dialectical components. The push–pulls of this process are ubiquitous and constantly shifting. What seemed appropriate and even necessary to disclose one day, or even one moment, may seem inopportune and inconceivable the next. The gratification and pride that followed the discussion of intimate material one day may turn to doubt and shame the next day. Conversely, the lack of trust that inhibited disclosure a moment ago may be replaced by a sense of intimacy that allows disclosure of long-suppressed thoughts or typically unexpressed personal feelings toward the other in the room. What is clear from reviewing various theoretical, research, and clinical perspectives on disclosure in psychotherapy is how complex this phenomenon really is. What follows is a synopsis of several of the more intricate aspects and dilemmas of disclosure among patients, therapists, supervisors, and supervisees.

THE CHOICE OF WHAT TO REVEAL

As has been noted throughout these pages, this fundamental issue is virtually always present in interpersonal situations and is rendered especially salient by the demand characteristics of the psychotherapeutic and supervisory settings. Many poets, novelists, and therapists have, in their own ways, noted that we never quite tell all and that we all die to a great extent unknown. In the songwriter Billy Joel's words (in "The Stranger"), "Though we share so many secrets, there are some we never tell."

But even posing the issue this way is too simplistic. Secrets and nondisclosures are rarely all-or-nothing phenomena. That is, we usually decide, even in therapy or in supervision, to reveal partially. We let some aspects of ourselves be known almost completely, others moderately, others slightly, others not all. Despite Jourard's entreaty, individuals, including patients, cannot always be fully open to others. Conversely, despite Freud's rule, therapists cannot be anonymous and unrevealing of themselves to their patients. Despite their desire to expose their work honestly and entirely, supervisees will sometimes emphasize their successes and minimize their errors. And, despite their wanting to present themselves as real and fallible, supervisors will sometimes present themselves as more knowledgeable and confident than they are truly feeling. Moreover, the proportion of what is shared about any topic changes dramatically depending upon who is sitting in the opposite chair. To some clients, I am quite revealing; to others, barely at all. Some clients have chosen to tell me parts of their stories that they could not tell to previous therapists, and I am sure that other clients have hidden aspects of themselves from me that they allowed other therapists to know.

Part of my task as a therapist and supervisor is to provide a safe enough place for disclosures. A related task is to expand the domain of what is considered by patients and supervisees as appropriate material to disclose. "My job," says the psychologist in Robertson Davies' book *The*

Manticore (1972), "is to listen to people say things they very badly want to tell but are afraid nobody else will understand" (p. 13).

We often titrate what we reveal. We check out our own emotional state as we are revealing, and we also evaluate how our words are being received. We may start intending to say little to our supervisor or therapist but find we are being heard well, far better than anticipated, and we reveal more and more. Or, we begin telling a supervisee a personally revealing anecdote but stop ourselves short, feeling awkward and too vulnerable. It is easy to forget that sometimes we are all more fragile than otherwise. In this vein, Kelly's (1998, 2000) emphasis on the benefits of repression in therapy is flawed because it ignores the fact that both patients and therapists monitor how much openness they can tolerate at any moment.

Related to the issue of what to reveal is the issue of to whom to reveal it. Some clients regard me as the person to whom they tell their most private stories, but others designate their spouse or best friend for this role. For this latter group of clients, I am primarily there to problem-solve, not to be privy to their secrets or to their feelings about me. In an episode of *Sex and the City*, one of the protagonists is asked, "Did you tell your therapist about it?" "Oh," she replies, "I couldn't possibly tell him. That's much too private." It is also sometimes easy to forget how artificial a setting therapy (or supervision) is, what a small slice of life gets shared. Clients and supervisees, for example, may disclose the most profound, intimate aspects of their lives but share little of their day-to-day activities. In this way, clients' friends and family often know far more about them than do their therapists. Omissions abound in therapy and supervision. In Woody Allen's movie *Deconstructing Harry*, a friend says to Harry: "You can't fool me. I'm not like your shrink. He only knows what you tell him. I know the truth."

Also related to the issue of what we disclose is how we disclose. Content does not define the entire domain of disclosure. What is the emotional relationship of the discloser to the disclosee as he or she is revealing something of importance? What is the relationship of the discloser to the material he or she is revealing? Among others, Wilhelm Reich (1949) drew our attention to the fact that *how* we say things is as important to understand as the content of what that we are saying.

We all construct our identities. We all have parts of ourselves that we like to feature in our self-presentation and "shadows" (Jung) that we strive to deny. We are all a combination of honest or semihonest reporting and self-serving storytelling, of various degrees of revealing and concealing. Our selves partly consist of the compromises we make between these contrasting states. These compromises, born of the ever-present conflict between disclosure and self-concealment, inevitably play out in psychotherapy and supervisory situations. What, how, and to whom we reveal remain fundamental and critical questions for all participants in the mental health field.

THE DIFFICULTY IN MAKING OURSELVES CLEAR

Following the question of "What am I willing to let another know about me?" lurks another critical question: "How do I adequately represent in words that which I am feeling and thinking?" Flaubert's words from Madame Bovary (cited at the beginning of this chapter) speak to the extraordinary difficulty we experience in attempting to translate what is in our minds to speech that is clear to ourselves and another. A similar thought was expressed by the Nobel Prize-winning Portuguese author Jose Saramago: "Human vocabulary is still not capable, and probably never will be, of knowing, recognizing, and communicating everything that can be humanly experienced and felt" (2002, p. 264). So, rarely is there direct correspondence between experience and words. So much is so often lost. I think of Woody Allen's absurd attempt at bending language to reflect a deeply held feeling. "I don't just love you," he says to Diane Keaton in *Annie Hall*, "I lurve you." Sometimes, too, our words and phrases are clear to ourselves but not to our listener. We struggle to find a common vocabulary and shared meanings of words. There are those (e.g., Derrida) who espouse even more extreme positions, contending that language distorts and opposes truth, that it is an impermeable boundary between ourselves and what is real.

Thus, even when patients (or therapists, etc.) are highly motivated to disclose a highly personal thought or feeling, they may feel they are failing at the task. Their words may sound hollow to them, missing the essence of what they are experiencing and want to share. Conversely, their words may sound clear and reasonably authentic to them but almost unintelligible to their listener, a situation that frustrates psychotherapeutic dyads (and even more so, spouses). We miss each other so often, even when we are highly motivated not to. One of the great contributions of Carl Rogers was his insistence on making sure that he understood what his client was trying to convey. Although frequently satirized as "echoing" his clients' words, Rogers was, instead, checking his understanding. He understood how difficult it often is for clients to clearly articulate what they are feeling, and how important it is for therapists to keep trying, again and again if necessary, to hear what clients mean to say. The same could be said of other relationships in psychotherapy. Clients, for example, should continually strive to ensure that they understand what their therapist is suggesting or asking.

Finally, this whole issue of making our disclosures clear to others presupposes a strong motivation to do so. When this is in doubt—as it often is because a good deal of the time we are ambivalent about whether and to what extent we should be disclosing—making ourselves clear to patients, therapists, supervisors, or supervisees becomes a near-impossible task. These are those situations in which a great deal of patience and a greater degree of empathy (e.g., "it feels to me you're not sure whether you'd like to share this with me"; "you seem to be struggling to find the right words to express what you mean") is required of the listener. Nevertheless, even with these skills present in the room, ambivalent disclosures add another layer of complexity to an already multilayered phenomenon.

THE DIFFICULTY IN BALANCING CONTRADICTORY NEEDS AND EMOTIONS

We may decide what to reveal and even choose relatively straightforward words to do so, but this does not preclude feeling confused or inundated by the tangled web of emotions attendant to expressing private aspects of ourselves. Therapists, clients, supervisees, and supervisors are all subject to these feelings. Jonathan Franzen, in his highly touted novel *The Corrections* (2001), wrote of the "vicious bipolarity of shame, that rapid cycling between confession and concealment" (p. 320). He was right but limited in his observation. It is not just shame that waxes and wanes in the disclosure process but a variety of positive and negative emotions.

Farber et al. (2004) studied the feelings patients experience in the process of disclosing in psychotherapy. Their results indicated that shame and vulnerability can and do coexist with such positive emotions as relief, pride, and authenticity. The process seems to unfold in a complicated if somewhat logical manner: "Shame lessens as disclosure occurs but does not dissipate entirely; concomitantly, positive emotions . . . emerge in their own right, partially (though not entirely) eclipsing the experience of shame and vulnerability" (p. 344). Following disclosure, individuals experience a mix of positive and negative emotions, although positive emotions tend to predominate. Farber et al. also note, though, that it remains unclear "whether and how this mixture of emotions changes hours or days after intense disclosures" (p. 344). I assume that this complex mix of shifting emotions occurs for each participant in the psychotherapeutic or supervisory situations even if the specific timing or mix of emotions differs according to role. I also assume that there is a wide variation in the way these emotions are experienced by individuals. For example, patients who tend to be nondisclosing are more likely to primarily experience shame following disclosure, whereas those on the higher end of the disclosing continuum likely experience both shame and relief.

This complicated picture gets even more complex if we remember that nondisclosures can be broken down into several subcategories, including secrets, hidden reactions, things left unsaid, and overt distortions or lies. The point here is that within each of these subcategories the particular mix of emotions experienced at a given time is likely to differ from other types of nondisclosures. For example, disclosing previously hidden reactions to a therapist's interventions may actually feel less safe than disclosing a long-held secret. The reason is that the former type of disclosure is more interpersonally situated and relates to the here and now of the dyadic interaction. The mix of emotions during and following disclosures is also likely to differ as a function of role. Therapists who withhold their reactions to their patients assumedly experience this differently (e.g., with less guilt) than patients or supervisees who withhold their reactions.

Farber et al. (2004) reported an apparent contradiction in clients' attitudes toward disclosure in therapy. On the one hand, clients seem to hold to the position that disclosing is always better than withholding thoughts or feelings. On the other hand, they also seem to believe that at times it is acceptable "not to tell." We concluded that there is an "ineluctable tension between clients' awareness of the value of disclosure and their equally held conviction that this position cannot always be honored" (p. 345). Again, I strongly suspect that this is equally true of therapists, supervisors, and supervisees: that they strongly value disclosure, both personally and professionally, but they also understand that a host of personal and interpersonal factors may interfere with the unfettered expression of this belief. Again, disclosure is a complicated endeavor.

THE MULTIPLE CONSEQUENCES OF DISCLOSURE

In addition to experiencing contradictory emotions before, during, and following disclosure, individuals may encounter a number of personal consequences of their behavior. Chapters 1 and 2 discussed in some detail many of these potential outcomes. Positive ones included a stronger sense of identity, a more intimate connection with the listener, and a reduction in physical and emotional distress; negative outcomes included regret, greater distance from the listener, and increases in physical and emotional distress. The overarching point here is that disclosure-related changes—changes in physical and emotional states, changes in self-perceptions, changes in one's perceptions of others, changes in others' perceptions of you, and changes in actual relationships with others—are likely to be experienced in a far more intricate, difficult-to-assimilate manner than a simple enumeration of positive and negative consequences would suggest. Positive and negative outcomes don't balance each other out. Each outcome leaves residues that may be difficult to integrate with other outcomes. The supervisee who discloses more than she "intended" in response to her supervisor's questioning may experience a number of consequences of this action: an immediate increase in anxiety, a postsupervisory session decrease in anxiety, a stronger perception of herself as courageous and highly motivated but also limited in clinical skills, a renewed perception of her supervisor as aggressive but also a good listener, and an increase in her own disclosing behaving toward her peers. Taken together, these effects may leave her somewhat proud of herself but also somewhat shaken.

THE ENDURING CONSEQUENCES OF DISCLOSURE

The consequences of disclosure, for all involved in therapy and supervision, not only are complex and overlapping but may also be enduring. Certain actions in life, including intimate disclosures, are essentially irreversible. Disclosing certain secrets (e.g., that one has abused another or been abused; that one has attempted suicide) may forever change the way one thinks about oneself and may also change what others think. Patients or supervisees, or even therapists or supervisors who disclose assumedly shameful material about their past, may leave the session feeling proud of what they have done ("I can be honest with others") and may engender a great deal of enduring respect in the listener ("I really admire her courage"). Similarly, allowing the other member of the dyad to know exactly what one is thinking or feeling ("I really care about you"; "I respect you greatly"; "I enjoy our work together"; "I'm not comfortable with what just happened") affects both participants and the nature of the relationship. The closeness that often ensues following a disclosure remains part of that relationship and may change forever expectations about what one can and should experience in other nontherapy or nonsupervisory relationships.

Thirty years ago a supervisor told me that he admired my work and felt that I was well on my way toward becoming an outstanding therapist. I have never forgotten that remark and sometimes still invoke it when I'm feeling unsure about what I'm doing clinically. A former supervisee of mine came back to visit me 10 years after our work together and reminded me of an acknowledgment I'd made to her (and long ago forgotten)—that I had struggled early in my career with working with clients older than myself but that I was glad I stuck with it and hoped that she would do so also. She told me that it made a significant difference in her career path, and she regarded it as a vote of confidence in her ability to get better at working with this population. Former patients of mine—and this is true of virtually every therapist I know—have returned years later to note that some remark has stayed with them for years. One ex-patient of mine said: "You let me know that your father was ill, and I felt so respected by your trust in me."

Of course, tactless or harsh disclosures may leave an enduring mark of a very different sort. Recently, a student in my program reported tearfully that a supervisor shared his observation that she was not sufficiently psychologically minded for effective clinical work. This remark came fairly early in the year. It would be hard to imagine either of the participants in this exchange forgetting this disclosure for the balance of their time together—and perhaps much longer. What comes to mind here are the words of the novelist Jonathan Lethem (2000): "The legacy of disclosure remained with us, a ghostly bond" (p. 42). This anecdote is also reminiscent of Richard Ford's (1986) well-turned phrase that "too much truth can be worse than death, and last longer" (p. 139).

There are several other aspects of disclosure that make it so complex a phenomenon. For one, it is a recursive process; that is, disclosures are a function of previous disclosures, building on them, affected by the reactions (in oneself and others) that these disclosures have elicited. Moreover, this process of building on previous disclosures is decidedly nonlinear. One marginally negative reaction to a disclosure of mine may effectively nullify a pattern of increasingly intimate statements. A patient's "Why are you telling me this?" may inhibit a therapist's disclosure to this patient for quite a long time. When a supervisee's acknowledgement of a mistake gets met with a tacit rebuke, or even nonverbal disapproval (e.g., a slight grimace), that supervisee may become quite reluctant to disclose another clinical error.

Understanding the nature and process of disclosure is also complicated by the frequency and ease with which we shift between various selves. As some poets have noted (e.g., Milocz), it is so very difficult to remain one person. Applying the concept of multiple selves to the study of disclosure allows us to see more clearly how we shift in what we want to tell another based on our current sense of self (how we regard ourselves at any given moment) and, relatedly, our predominant mood (how we feel). A patient may declare early in one session that "I just don't feel like talking right now" and later that "I really need to share something important with you." There are days when therapists wake up (and come to work) feeling gloomy and closed; there are days when we're feeling exuberant and expansive. How we experience ourselves during a session (whether as a patient, therapist, supervisor, or supervisee) affects our tendency to disclose, some of which is surely affected by what occurs in session but some of which is also determined by events that occurred before a session has begun.

There is a burgeoning clinical and research literature on disclosure among patients, therapists, supervisors, and supervisees. At the same time, it is apparent that this is still a relatively unexplored topic with many unanswered questions. For example, the issue of matching specific therapist interventions to specific client needs, a topic of great contemporary interest in the psychotherapy research community, remains mostly unexplored in relationship to disclosure. Are certain therapist disclosures especially beneficial with clients with different diagnoses? Should the frequency or content of therapist disclosures differ when working with clients whose primary therapeutic goals are insight and growth as opposed to those whose goals are symptom reduction and immediate relief from distress?

Another issue that requires further empirical and clinical work: distinguishing differences in content, tone, and consequences between disclosures that are solicited and those that are spontaneous. Clients are likely to experience their disclosures one way when they have been prompted and quite another way when these statements have emerged more volitionally. The same is true for therapists, supervisors, and supervisees. Perhaps there are optimal levels of questioning in these situations—too little may leave valuable information unknown, too much or too aggressive questioning may result in constriction. Future work in the area might also focus on the issue of style. Self-disclosures are so influenced by personal style, and so little work has been done on this topic. How do we disclose nonverbally? What expressive movements accompany our verbal disclosures? What medium do we prefer to use to disclose? What nonverbal expressions are important to us when we are disclosed to? What media feel authorized in therapy or supervisory situations? The protagonist in Judith Rossner's (1983) book *August* used photographs of her family to disclose intense early childhood issues that were not communicable through words alone.

Most importantly, it remains unclear what the relationship is between therapist or patient disclosure and therapeutic outcome. Similarly, there are too few studies to draw firm conclusions regarding the relationship between supervisee or supervisor disclosure and either patient outcome or supervisee improvement. What seems most clear at this time is that, to be effective, disclosures must ultimately lead to new cognitive or emotional patterns of processing information. Still, far more research is necessary to understand how disclosures in therapy and supervision affect the participants on both a short-term and long-term basis.

Disclosure is so fundamentally a human process. Most of us have a strong need to feel known—one that is usually stronger, if only marginally, than our need to remain private and unknown. "I have discovered," wrote Walker Percy in his classic (1960) novel *The Moviegoer*, "that most people have no one to talk to, no one that is, who really wants to listen. When it does at least dawn on a man that you really want to hear about his business, the look that comes over his face is something to see" (p. 64). The therapist's or supervisor's office, symbols of confidentiality, serve as ideal laboratories for examining the ways in which individuals exert their needs to be known while simultaneously exerting their needs to be private and unknown, for testing the limits of personal openness, and for understanding the short and long-term consequences of disclosure.

Attempts at disclosure—even sincere, persistent attempts—may ultimately be near-misses at best. We are fallible as disclosers and equally fallible as listeners. But disclosures often succeed somewhat and with great consequence. Personal disclosures, especially in the safe confines of a therapist's office, represent a profound means to further our sense of self while enhancing our connection to important others. Here are some final thoughts on this issue, courtesy of "Grace," a particularly courageous patient of mine:

Self-Disclosure

Naked,
I stand before you,
Not discarding my robe,
But gently placing it
Near me,
Should I need it.

Baring
The splendor and the scars,
I disclose to you
An exposed self,
Freer to be
Among the living

References

Acosta, F. X., & Sheehan, J. G. (1978). Self-disclosure in relation to psychotherapist expertise and ethnicity. *American Journal of Community Psychology, 6*(6), 545–553.

Adler, J. (2002). *Offering from the conscious body: The discipline of authentic movement.* Rochester, VT: Inner Traditions International.

Adler, N. E., Boyce, T., Chesney, M. A., Cohen, S., Folkman, S., Kahn, R. L., et al. (1994). Socioeconomic status and health: The challenge of the gradient. *American Psychologist, 49,* 15–24.

Akamatsu, N. N. (1995). The defiant daughter and compliant mother: Multicultural dialogues on woman's role. *In Session: Psychotherapy in Practice, 1,* 43–55.

Al-Mateen, C. S. (1991). Simultaneous pregnancy in the therapist and patient. *American Journal of Psychotherapy, 45,* 432–444

Alonzo, A., & Ruttan, S. J. (1988). Shame and guilt in psychotherapy supervision. *Psychotherapy, 25,* 576–581.

Alvarez, M. (1999). Diversity among Latinas: Implications for college mental health. In Y. M. Jenkins (Ed.), *Diversity in college settings: Directives for helping professionals* (pp. 99–115). New York: Routledge.

American Psychological Association. (2002). Ethical principles of psychologists and code of conduct. *American Psychologist, 57,* 1060–1073.

Anchor, K. N., & Sandler, H. M. (1973). Psychotherapy sabotage and avoidance of self-disclosure. In *Proceedings of the Annual Convention of the American Psychological Association,* pp. 485–486. Washington, DC: American Psychological Association.

Anderson, S. C., & Mandell, D. L. (1989, May). The use of therapist self-disclosure by professional social workers. *Social Casework: The Journal for Contemporary Social Work, 70,* 259–267.

Anstadt, T., Merten, J., Ullrich, B., & Krause, R. (1997). Affective dyadic behavior, core conflictual relationship themes, and success of treatment. *Psychotherapy Research, 7,* 397–417.

Aron, L. (1991). The patient's experience of the analyst's subjectivity. *Psychoanalytic Dialogues, 1,* 29–51.

Aron, L. (1996). *A meeting of minds: Mutuality in psychoanalysis.* Hillsdale, NJ: Analytic Press.

Asai, A., & Barnlund, D. C. (1998). Boundaries of unconscious, private, and public self in Japanese and Americans: A cross-cultural comparison. *International Journal of Intercultural Relations, 22,* 31–52.

Atkinson, D. R., Brown, M. T., Parham, T. A., Matthews, L. G., Landrum-Brown, J., & Kim, A. U. (1996). African American client skin tone and clinical judgments of African American and European American psychologists. *Professional Psychology: Research and Practice, 27,* 500–505.

Atkinson, D. R., & Gim, R. H. (1989). Asian-American cultural identity and attitudes toward mental health services. *Journal of Counseling Psychology, 36,* 209–212.

Atkinson, D. R., Morten, G., & Sue, D. W. (1998). *Counseling American minorities* (5th ed.). New York: McGraw-Hill.

Audet, C., & Everall, R. D. (2003). Counsellor self-disclosure: Client-informed implications for practice. *Counselling and Psychotherapy Research, 3,* 223–231.

Bachelor, A. (1995). Clients' perception of the therapeutic alliance: A qualitative analysis. *Journal of Counseling Psychology, 42,* 323–337.

Bair, D. (2003). *Jung: A biography.* New York: Little, Brown.

Ball, J. (1999). Identity formation in Confucian heritage societies: Implications for theory, research, and practice. In P. Peterson (Ed.), *Multiculturalism as a fourth force* (pp. 147–165). Philadelphia: Brunner/Mazel.

Barish, K. (2004). The child therapist's generative use of self. *Journal of Infant, Child, and Adolescent Psychotherapy, 3,* 270–282.

Barnlund, D. G. (1975). *Public and private self in Japan and the United States.* Portland, OR: Intercultural Press.

Barnlund, D. G. (1989). *Communicative styles of Japanese and Americans: Images and realities.* Belmont, CA: Wadsworth.

Barrett, M. S., & Berman, J. S. (2001). Is psychotherapy more effective when therapists disclose information about themselves? *Journal of Consulting and Clinical Psychology, 69,* 597–603.

Basescu, S. (1977). Anxieties in the analyst: An autobiographical account. In K. A. Frank (Ed.), *The human dimension in psychoanalytic practice* (pp. 153–163). New York: Grune & Stratton.

Basescu, S. (1987). Behind the "scenes": The inner experience of at least one psychoanalyst. *Psychoanalytic Psychology, 4,* 255–265.

Basescu, S. (1990). Show and tell: Reflections on the analyst's self-disclosure. In G. Stricker & M. Fisher (Eds.), *Self-disclosure in the therapeutic relationship* (pp. 47–59). New York: Plenum Press.

Bass, E., & Davis, L. (1988). *The courage to heal: A guide for women survivors of child sexual abuse.* New York: Harper & Row.

Beck, A., Freeman, A., & Associates (1990). *Cognitive therapy of personality disorders.* New York: Guilford Press.

Becker, E. (1973). *The denial of death.* New York: Free Press.

Bellow, S. (1982). *The dean's December.* New York: Harper & Row.

Benjamin, J. (1988). *The bonds of love.* New York: Pantheon Books.

Benjamin, J. (1992). Recognition and destruction: An outline of intersubjectivity. In N. Skolnick & S. Warshaw (Eds.), *Relational perspectives in psychoanalysis* (pp. 43–60). Hillsdale, NJ: Analytic Press.

Benjamin, J. (1994). What angel would hear me?: The erotics of transference. *Psychoanalytic Inquiry, 14*, 535–557.

Benjamin, J. (1998). *Shadow of the other.* New York: Routledge.

Bennun, I., & Schindler, L. (1988). Therapist and patient factors in the behavioural treatment of phobic patients. *Journal of Clinical Psychology, 27*, 145–150.

Berano, K., & Farber, B. A. (2006, June). *Asian-American and Caucasian self-disclosure in psychotherapy.* Paper presented at the annual meeting of the Society for Psychotherapy Research, Edinburgh, Scotland.

Berg, I. K., & Jaya, A. (1993). Different and same: Family therapy with Asian-American families. *Journal of Marital and Family Therapy, 19*, 31–38.

Berg-Cross, L. (1984). Therapist self-disclosure to clients in psychotherapy. *Psychotherapy in Private Practice, 2*, 57–64.

Bersoff, D. N. (1976). Therapists as protectors and policemen: New roles as a result of Tarasoff? In D. N. Bersoff (Ed.). *Ethical conflicts in psychology* (3rd ed., pp. 165–166, 2003). Washington, DC: American Psychological Association.

Beutler, L. E., & Mitchell, R. (1981). Differential psychotherapy outcome among depressed and impulsive patients as a function of analytic and experiential treatment procedures. *Psychiatry: Journal for the Study of Interpersonal Processes, 44*, 297–306.

Beutler, L. E., Moleiro, C., & Talebi, H. (2002). Resistance in psychotherapy: What conclusions are supported by research? *Journal of Clinical Psychology, 58*, 207–217.

Block, L. (1991). Keller's therapy. In E. Kates (Ed.), *On the couch: Great American stories about therapy* (pp. 123–155). New York: Atlantic Monthly Press, 1997.

Bloom, A. (1993). Psychoanalysis changed my life. In E. Kates (Ed.), *On the couch: Great American stories about therapy.* New York: Atlantic Monthly Press, 1997.

Blustein, D. L. (1994). Who am I?: The question of self and identity in career development. In M. L. Savickas & R. W. Lent (Eds.), *Convergence in career development theories* (pp. 139–154). Palo Alto, CA: Consulting Psychologists Press.

Blustein, D. L., & Nourmair, D. A. (1996). Self and identity in career development: Implications for theory and practice. *Journal of Counseling and Development, 74*, 433–441.

Bonanno, G. A. (2004). Loss, trauma, and human resilience: Have we underestimated the human capacity to thrive after extremely aversive events? *American Psychologist, 59*, 20–28.

Bonanno, G. A., Keltner, D., Holen, A., & Horowitz, M. J. (1995). When avoiding unpleasant emotions might not be such a bad thing: Verbal autonomic response dissociation and midlife conjugal bereavement. *Journal of Personality and Social Psychology, 69*, 975–989.

Bonanno, G. A., Keltner, D., Noll, J. G., Putnam, F. W., Trickett, P. K., Lejeune, J., et al. (2002). When the face reveals what words do not: Facial expressions of emotion, smiling, and the willingness to disclose childhood sexual abuse. *Journal of Personality and Social Psychology, 83*, 94–110.

Bonanno, G. A., Papa, A., O'Neill, K., Westphal, M., & Coifman, K. (2004). The importance of being flexible: The ability to both enhance and suppress emotional expression predicts long-term adjustment. *Psychological Science, 15*, 482–487.

Bootzin, R. R. (1997). Examining the theory and clinical utility of writing about emotional experiences. *Psychological Science, 8*, 167–169.

Borkovec, T. D., Roemer, L., & Kenyon, J. (1995). Disclosure and worry: Opposite sides of the emotional processing coin. In J. W. Pennebaker (Ed.), *Emotion, disclosure, and health* (pp. 47–70). Washington, DC: American Psychological Association.

Borys, D. S., & Pope, K. S. (1989). Dual relationships between therapist and client: A national study of psychologists, psychiatrists, and social workers. *Professional Psychology: Research and Practice, 20*, 283–293.

Bradshaw, C. K. (1994). Asian and Asian American women: Historical and political considerations in psychotherapy. In L. Comas-Diaz & B. Greene (Eds.), *Women of color* (pp. 72–113). New York: Guilford Press.

Braswell, L., Kendall, P. C., Braith, J., Carey, M. P., & Vye, C. S. (1985). "Involvement" in cognitive behavioral therapy with children: Process and its relationship to outcome. *Cognitive Therapy and Research, 9*, 611–630.

Bridges, N. A. (2001). Therapist self-disclosure: Expanding the comfort zone. *Psychotherapy, 38*, 21–30.

Brock, G. (1987). *Ethics casebook*. Washington, DC: American Association for Marriage and Family Therapy.

Bromberg, P. (1994). "Speak! That I may see you": Some reflections on dissociation, reality, and psychoanalytic listening. *Psychoanalytic Dialogues, 4*, 517–547.

Broucek, F. J. (1991). *Same and the self*. New York: Guilford Press.

Brunswick, R. M. (1928). A supplement to Freud's "History of an Infantile Neurosis." *International Journal of Psycho-Analysis, 9*, 439–476.

Bucci, W. (1997). *Psychoanalysis and cognitive science: A multiple code theory*. New York: Guilford Press.

Bullitt, C., & Farber, B. A. (2002). Sex differences in the relationship between interpersonal problems and defensive style. *Psychological Reports, 91*, 767–768.

Busch, F. (1998). Self-disclosure ain't what it's cracked up to be, at least not yet. *Psychoanalytic Inquiry, 18*, 518–529.

Capobianco, J., & Farber, B. A. (2005). Therapist self-disclosure to child patients. *American Journal of Psychotherapy, 59*, 199–212.

Carter, R. T. (1991). Cultural values: A review of empirical research and implications for counseling. *Journal of Counseling and Development, 70*, 164–173.

Cerbone, A. R. (1991). The effects of political activism on psychotherapy: A case study. In C. Silverstein (Ed.), *Gays, lesbians, and their therapists* (pp. 40–51). New York: Norton.

Chapa, J., & Valencia, R. (1993). Latino population growth, demographic characteristics, and educational stagnation: An examination of recent trends. *Latino Journal of Behavioral Sciences, 15*, 165–187.

Chelune, G. J. (1979). Measuring openness in interpersonal communication. In G. J. Chelune & Associates (Eds.), *Self-disclosure: Origins, patterns and implications of openness in interpersonal relationships* (pp. 1–27). San Francisco: Jossey-Bass.

Chen, G. M. (1995). Differences in self-disclosure patterns among Americans versus Chinese: A comparative study. *Journal of Cross-Cultural Psychology, 26*, 84–91.

Cherbosque, J. (1987). Differential effects of counselor self-disclosure statements on perception of the counselor and willingness to disclose: A cross-cultural study. *Psychotherapy, 24*, 434–437.

Chethik, M. (2000). *Techniques of child therapy: Psychodynamic strategies* (2nd ed.). New York: Guilford Press.

Chiaramonte, J. A. (1986). Therapist pregnancy and maternity leave: Maintaining and furthering therapeutic gains in the interim. *Clinical Social Work Journal, 14,* 335–348.

Chu, S. H. (1999). Multi-cultural counseling: An Asian-American perspective. In D. S. Sandhu (Ed.), *Asian and Pacific Islander Americans: Issues and concerns for counseling and psychotherapy* (pp. 21–30). New York: Nova Science.

Chung, R. C., Bemak, F., & Kilinc, A. (2002). Culture and empathy: Case studies in cross-cultural counseling. In P. R. Breggin & G. Breggin (Eds.), *Dimensions of empathic therapy* (pp. 119–128). New York: Springer.

Clarkson, S. E. (1980). Pregnancy as a transference stimulus. *British Journal of Medical Psychology, 53,* 313–317.

Coates, D., & Winston, T. (1987). The dilemma of stress disclosure. In V. J. Derlega & J. H. Berg (Eds.), *Self-disclosure: Theory, research, and therapy* (pp. 229–255). New York: Plenum Press.

Collins, N. L., & Miller, L. C. (1994). Self-disclosure and liking: A meta-analytic review. *Psychological Bulletin, 116,* 457–475.

Comas-Diaz, L., & Greene, B. (1994). Overview: An ethnocultural mosaic. In L. Comas-Diaz & B. Greene (Eds.), *Women of color* (pp. 3–9). New York: Guilford Press.

Constantine, M. G., & Gloria, A. M. (1999). Multicultural issues in predoctoral internship programs: A national survey. *Journal of Multicultural Counseling Development, 27,* 4–53.

Constantine, M. G., & Kwan, K. L. (2003). Cross-cultural considerations of therapist self-disclosure. *Journal of Clinical Psychology, 59,* 581–588.

Costin, C., & Johnson, C. L. (2002). Been there, done that: Clinicians' use of personal recovery in the treatment of eating disorders. *Eating Disorders, 10,* 293–303.

Counselman, E. F., & Alonso, A. (1993). The ill therapist: therapists' reactions to personal illness and its impact on psychotherapy. *American Journal of Psychotherapy, 47,* 591–602.

Cozby, P. C. (1973). Self-disclosure: A literature review. *Psychological Bulletin, 79,* 73–91.

Crews, F. (1984, June). The Freudian way of knowledge. *The New Criterion, 3,* 7–25.

Curtis, R., Field, C., Knaan-Kostman, I., & Mannix, K. (2004). What 75 psychoanalysts found helpful and hurtful in their own analyses. *Psychoanalytic Psychology, 21,* 183–202.

Davies, R. (1972). *The Manticore.* New York: Penguin Books.

DeLillo, D. (1985). *White noise.* New York: Penguin Books.

Derlega, V. J., Metts, S., Petronio, S., & Margulis, S. T. (1993). *Self-disclosure.* Newbury Park, CA: Sage.

Derlega, V. J., Lovell, R., & Chaikin, A. L. (1976). Effects of therapist disclosure and its perceived appropriateness on client self-disclosure. *Journal of Consulting and Clinical Psychology, 44,* 866.

Dindia, K., & Allen, M. (1992). Sex differences in self-disclosure: A meta-analysis. *Psychological Bulletin, 112,* 106–124.

Dixon, L., Adler, D., Braun, D., Dulit, R., Goldman, B., Siris, S., et al. (2001). Reexamination of therapist self-disclosure. *Psychiatric Services, 52,* 1489–1493.

Domanico, Y. B., Crawford, I., & Wolfe, A. S. (1994). Ethnic identity and self-concept in Mexican-American adolescents: Is bicultural identity related to stress or better adjustment? *Child and Youth Care Forum, 23,* 197–207.

Dostoyevsky, F. (1868). *The idiot.* New York: Modern Library, 1935.

Drescher, J. (2002). Don't ask, don't tell: A gay man's perspective on the psychoanalytic training experience between 1973 and 1991. *Journal of Gay and Lesbian Psychotherapy, 6,* 45–55.

Dryden, W. (1990). Self-disclosure in rational-emotive therapy. In G. Stricker & M. Fisher (Eds.), *Self-disclosure in the therapeutic relationship* (pp. 61–74). New York: Plenum Press.

Dupont, J. (1988). Introduction. In J. Dupont (Ed.), *The clinical diary of Sandor Ferenczi* (pp. xi–xxvii). Cambridge, MA: Harvard University Press.

Durban, J., Lazar, R., & Ofer, G. (1993). The cracked container, the containing crack: Chronic illness–its effects on the therapist and the therapeutic process. *International Journal of Psycho-Analysis, 74,* 705–713.

Eco, U. (1996). *The island of the day before.* New York: Penguin Books.

Edwards, C. E., & Murdock, N. L. (1994). Characteristics of therapist self-disclosure in the counseling process. *Journal of Counseling and Development, 72,* 384–389.

Ekman, P., & Rosenberg, E. (Eds.). (1998). *What the face reveals: Basic and applied studies of spontaneous expression using the facial action coding system.* New York: Oxford University Press.

Ellenberger, H. F. (1970). *The discovery of the unconscious: The history and evolution of dynamic psychiatry.* New York: Basic Books.

Engle, D., & Holiman, M. (2002). A Gestalt–experiential perspective on resistance. *Journal of Clinical Psychology, 58,* 175–183.

Epstein, L. (1995). Self-disclosure and analytic space. *Contemporary Psychoanalysis, 31,* 229–236.

Epstein, R. S. (1994). *Keeping boundaries: Maintaining safety and integrity in the psychotherapeutic process.* Washington, DC: American Psychiatric Press.

Etchegoyen, R. H. (1991). *The fundamentals of psychoanalytic technique.* London: Karnac Books.

Everstine, L., Everstine, D. S., Heymann, G. M., True, R. H., Frey, D. H., Johnson, H. G., et al. (1980). Privacy and confidentiality in psychotherapy. In D. N. Bersoff (Ed.), *Ethical conflicts in psychology* (3rd ed., pp. 162–164). Washington, DC: American Psychological Association.

Fairbairn, W. R. D. (1946). Object-relationships and dynamic structure. *International Journal of Psycho-Analysis, 27,* 30–37.

Falicov, C. J. (1998). *Latino families in therapy: A guide to multicultural practice.* New York: Guilford Press.

Fang, S. S., & Wark, L. (1998). Developing cross-cultural competence with traditional Chinese Americans in family therapy: Background information and the initial therapeutic contact. *Contemporary Family Therapy, 20,* 59–77.

Farber, B. A. (1989). Psychological-mindedness: Can there be too much of a good thing? *Psychotherapy, 26,* 210–217.

Farber, B. A. (2003). Patient self-disclosure: A review of the research. *Journal of Clinical Psychology, 59,* 589–600.

Farber, B. A., Berano, K. C., & Capobianco, J. A. (2004). Clients' perceptions of the process and consequences of self-disclosure in psychotherapy. *Journal of Counseling Psychology, 51,* 340–346.

Farber, B. A., Brink, D., & Raskin, P. (Eds.). (1996). *The psychotherapy of Carl Rogers: Cases and commentary.* New York: Guilford Press.

Farber, B. A., & Hall, D. (1992). *Disclosure to therapists: What is and is not discussed in therapy.* Paper presented at the annual meeting of the Society for Psychotherapy Research, Berkeley, CA.

Farber, B. A., & Hall, D. (2002). Disclosure to therapists: What is and is not discussed in psychotherapy. *Journal of Clinical Psychology, 58,* 359–370.

Farber, B. A., & Lane, J. S. (2002). Effective elements of the therapy relationship: Positive regard. In J. Norcross (Ed.), *Psychotherapy relationships that work: Therapist contributions and responsiveness to patients* (pp. 175–194). New York: Oxford University Press.

Farber, B. A., & Sohn, A. (1997, August). *Patient disclosure and denial: A delicate balance.* Paper presented at the annual meeting of the American Psychological Association, Chicago, IL.

Farber, B. A., & Sohn, A. (2001, June). *The relationship of patient disclosure to therapy outcome.* Paper presented at the annual meeting of the Society for Psychotherapy Research, Montevideo, Uruguay.

Ferenczi, S. (1926). *Further contributions to the theory and technique of psychoanalysis.* Honolulu, HI: Hogarth Press.

Ferenczi, S. (1932). *Clinical diary* (J. Dupont, Ed., M. Balint & N. Zarday Jackson, Trans.). Cambridge, MA: Harvard University Press, 1988.

Ferenczi, S. (1933). Confusion of tongues between adults and the child (E. Mosbacher, Trans.). In M. Balint (Ed.), *Final contributions to the problems and methods of psycho-analysis* (pp. 156–157). New York: Basic Books, 1955.

Flaubert, G. (1856) *Madame Bovary* (F. Steegmuller, Trans.). New York: Modern Library, 1992.

Folkman, S., & Lazarus, R. S. (1988). Coping as a mediator of emotion. *Journal of Personality and Social Psychology, 54,* 466–475.

Ford, R. (1986). *The sportswriter.* New York: Vintage Books.

Fosha, D. (2000). *The transforming power of affect: A model for accelerated change.* New York: Basic Books.

Fosha, D. (2004, February 17). *Short term dynamic therapy discussion list.* Message posted to electronic mailing list, STDP-List@stdp.org.

Franco, J. N., Malloy, T., & Gonzalez, R. (1984). Ethnic and acculturation differences in self-disclosure. *Journal of Social Psychology, 122,* 21–32.

Frank, J. D. (1974). *Persuasion and healing: A comparative study of psychotherapy* (rev. ed.). New York: Schocken Books.

Frankl, V. E. (1997). *Man's search for meaning* (rev. ed.). New York: Pocket Books.

Franzen, J. (2001). *The corrections.* New York: Picardo.

Freedman, S. R., & Enright, R. D. (1996). Forgiveness as an intervention goal with incest survivors. *Journal of Consulting and Clinical Psychology, 64,* 155–176.

Freud, A. (1958). Adolescence. *Psychoanalytic Study of the Child, 13,* 255–278.

Freud, S. (1905). Fragment of an analysis of a case of hysteria, Dora: The first dream. In P. Gay (Ed.), *The Freud reader* (pp. 172–238). New York: Norton, 1989.

Freud, S. (1912). Recommendations to physicians practicing psychoanalysis. In J. Strachey (Ed. & Trans.), *The standard edition of the complete psychological works of Sigmund Freud* (Vol. 12, pp. 109–120). London: Hogarth Press, 1966.

Freud, S. (1913). On beginning the treatment. In J. Strachey (Ed. & Trans.), *The standard edition of the complete psychological works of Sigmund Freud* (Vol. 12, pp. 121–144). London: Hogarth Press, 1958.

Friedman, G. (1991). Impact of a therapist's life threatening illness on the therapeutic situation. *Contemporary Psychoanalysis, 27*, 405–421.

Fromm-Reichmann, F. (1952). Personality of the psychotherapist and the doctor–patient relationship. In D. M. Bullard (Ed.), *Psychoanalysis and psychotherapy: Selected papers of Frieda Fromm-Reichmann* (pp. 100–104). Chicago: University of Chicago Press, 1959.

Frum, D. (2000). *How we got here: The 70s: The decade that brought you modern life—for better or worse.* New York: Basic Books.

Fuller Stockman, A., & Green-Emrich, A. (1994). Impact of therapist pregnancy on the process of counseling and psychotherapy. *Psychotherapy: Theory, Research, Practice, Training, 31*, 456–462.

Gabbard, G. O., & Lester, E. P. (1995). *Boundaries and boundary violations in psychoanalysis.* New York: Basic Books.

Gaines, R. (2003). Therapist self-disclosure with children, adolescents, and their parents. *Journal of Clinical Psychology in Session, 59*, 589–588.

Gardner, R. A. (1993). *Psychotherapy with children.* Northvale, NJ: Aronson.

Gartrell, N. (1984). *Colloquium: Issues in psychotherapy with lesbian women.* Wellesley, MA: Wellesley College, Stone Center for Developmental Services and Studies.

Gay, P. (1989). *Freud: A life for our time.* New York: Norton.

Geller, J. D. (1994). The psychotherapist's experience of interest and boredom. *Psychotherapy, 31*, 3–16.

Geller, J. D. (2001, June). *The case for therapist disclosure: Differences in working with mental health professionals versus non-professionals.* Paper presented at the annual meeting of the Society for Psychotherapy Research, Montevideo, Uruguay.

Geller, J. D. (2005a). Boundaries and internalization in the psychotherapy of psychotherapists. In J. D. Geller, J. C. Norcross, & D. E. Orlinsky (Eds.), *The psychotherapist's own psychotherapy: Patient and clinician perspectives* (pp. 379–404). New York: Oxford University Press.

Geller, J. D. (2005b). Style and its contribution to a patient-specific mode of therapeutic technique. *Psychotherapy: Theory, Research, Practice, Training, 42*, 469–483.

Geller, J. D., Cooley, R. S., & Hartley, D. (1982). Images of the psychotherapist: A theoretical and methodological perspective. *Imagination, Cognition and Personality, 1*, 123–146.

Geller, J. D., & Farber, B. A. (1993). Factors influencing the process of internalization in psychotherapy. *Psychotherapy Research, 3*, 166–180.

Geller, J. D., & Farber, B. A. (1997, August). *What therapists do and don't tell their patients.* Paper presented at the annual meeting of the American Psychological Association, Chicago.

Gergen, K. (1985). The social constructionist movement in modern psychology. *American Psychologist, 40,* 266–275.

Gerson, S. (1996). Neutrality, resistance, and self-disclosure in an intersubjective psychoanalysis. *Psychoanalytic Dialogues, 6,* 623–645.

Ginzberg, K., Solomon, Z., & Bleich, A. (2002). Repressive coping style, acute stress disorder, and posttraumatic stress disorder after myocardial infarction. *Psychosomatic Medicine, 64,* 748–757.

Glosoff, H. L., Herlihy, S. B., Herlihy, B., & Spence, E. B. (1997). Privileged communication in the psychologist–client relationship. *Professional Psychology: Research and Practice, 28,* 573–581.

Goffman, E. (1959). *The presentation of self in everyday life.* Garden City, NY: Doubleday.

Goldfried, M. R., Burckell, L. A., & Eubanks-Carter, C. (2003). Therapist self-disclosure in cognitive-behavior therapy. *Journal of Clinical Psychology/In Session, 59,* 555–568.

Goldstein, E. G. (1994). Self-disclosure in treatment: What therapists do and don't talk about. *Clinical Social Work Journal, 22,* 417–433.

Goldstein, E. G. (1997). To tell or not to tell: The disclosure of events in the therapist's life to the patient. *Clinical Social Work Journal, 25,* 41–58.

Greben, S. E., & Ruskin, R. (1994). Introduction: Significant aspects of the supervisor–supervisee relationship and interaction. In S. E. Greben & R. Ruskin (Eds.), *Clinical perspectives on psychotherapy supervision* (pp. 1–10). Washington, DC: American Psychiatric Press.

Greenberg, J., & Cheselka, O. (1995). Relational approaches to psychoanalytic psychotherapy. In A. S. Gurman & S. B. Messer (Eds.), *Essential psychotherapies: Theory and practice.* New York: Aronson.

Greenberg, J. R., & Mitchell, S. A. (1983). *Object relations in psychoanalytic theory.* Cambridge, MA: Harvard University Press.

Greene, B. (1994). African American women. In L. Comas-Díaz & B. Greene (Eds.), *Women of color* (pp. 10–29). New York: Guilford Press.

Grier, W., & Cobbs, P. (1968). *Black rage.* New York: Bantam Books.

Groddeck, G. (1923). *The book of the it.* London: Vision Press, 1950.

Grubrich-Simitis, I. (1986). Six letters of Sigmund Freud and Sandor Ferenczi on the interrelationship of psychoanalytic theory and technique. *International Review of Psycho-Analysis, 13,* 259–277.

Guntrip, H. (1961). *Personality structure and human interaction: The developing synthesis of psycho-dynamic theory.* New York: International Universities Press.

Guntrip, H. (1975). My experience of analysis with Fairbairn and Winnicott. *International Review of Psycho-Analysis, 2,* 145–156.

Gussow, M. (1998, April 28). A novelist builds out from fact to reach the truth: John Irving begins with his memories. *The New York Times,* pp. E1, E6.

Haber, S. (1992). Women in independent practice: Issues of pregnancy and motherhood. *Psychotherapy in Private Practice, 11,* 25–29.

Hahn, W. K. (2001). The experience of shame in psychotherapy supervision. *Psychotherapy: Theory, Research, Practice, Training, 38,* 272–282.

Hall, D. A., & Farber, B. A. (2001). Patterns of patient disclosure in psychotherapy. *Journal of the American Academy of Psychoanalysis, 29,* 213–230.

Hall, E. T. (1976). *Beyond culture.* New York: Doubleday.

Halpert, E. (1982). When the analyst is chronically ill or dying. *Psychoanalytic Quarterly, 51*, 372–389.

Ham, D. C. (1993). Empathy. In J. L. Chin (Ed.), *Transference and empathy in Asian Americans psychotherapy: Cultural values and treatment needs* (pp. 35–62). Westport, CT: Praeger.

Hanly, C. (1998). Reflections on the analyst's self-disclosure. *Psychoanalytic Inquiry, 18*, 550–565.

Harrison, J. (2004, November 21). The poetry symposium. *The New York Times Book Review*, pp. 10, 13–15.

Haut, M. W., & Muehleman, T. (1986). Informed consent: The effects of clarity and specificity on disclosure in a clinical interview. *Psychotherapy: Theory, Research, Practice, Training, 23*, 93–101.

Hessling, R. S., & Kahn, J. H. (2000). *A longitudinal study of change in relational schemas.* Unpublished manuscript, Iowa State University, Ames.

Hill, C. E. (1989). *Therapist techniques and client outcomes: Eight cases of brief psychotherapy.* Newbury Park, CA: Sage.

Hill, C. E., Gelso, C. J., & Mohr, J. J. (2000). Client concealment and self-presentation in therapy: Comment on Kelly (2000). *Psychological Bulletin, 126*, 495–500.

Hill, C. E., Helms, J. E., Tichenor, V., Spiegel, S. B., O'Grady, K. E., & Perry, E. S. (1988). Effects of therapist response modes in brief psychotherapy. *Journal of Counseling Psychology, 35*, 222–233.

Hill, C. E., & Knox, S. (2002). Self-disclosure. In J. Norcross (Ed.), *Psychotherapy relationships that work: Therapist contributions and responsiveness to patients* (pp. 255–265). New York: Oxford University Press.

Hill, C. E., Mahalik, J. R., & Thompson, B. J. (1989). Therapist self-disclosure. *Psychotherapy: Theory, Research, Practice, Training, 26*, 290–295.

Hill, C. E., & O'Brien, K. M. (1999). Self-disclosure. In C. E. Hill & K. M. O'Brien (Eds.), *Helping skills: Facilitating exploration, insight, and action* (pp. 223–234). Washington, DC: American Psychological Association.

Hill, C. E., Thompson, B. J., Cogar, M., & Denman, D. W. (1993). Beneath the surface of long-term therapy: Therapist and client reports of their own and each other's covert processes. *Journal of Counseling Psychology, 40*, 278–287.

Hill, C. E., Thompson, B. J., & Corbett, M. M. (1992). The impact of therapist ability to perceive displayed and hidden client reactions on immediate outcome in first sessions of brief therapy. *Psychotherapy Research, 2*, 143–155.

Hoffman, M. A., Hill, C. E., Holmes, S. E., & Freitas, G. F. (2005). Supervisor perspective on the process and outcome of giving easy, difficult, or no feedback to supervisees. *Journal of Counseling Psychology, 52*, 3–13.

Hoffman, M. A., & Spencer, G. P. (1977). Effect of interviewer self-disclosure and interviewer–subject sex pairing on perceived and actual subject behavior. *Journal of Counseling Psychology, 24*, 383–390.

Hohenadel, K. (2004, March 14). Breaking France's final taboo: Filming sex isn't dirty but making movies about money is. *The New York Times, Arts and Leisure*, p. 13.

Holzer, C. E., Goldsmith, H. F., & Ciarlo, J. A. (1998). Effects of rural–urban county type on the availability of health and mental health care providers. In

R. W. Manderscheid & M. J. Henderson (Eds.), *Mental health, United States*. Rockville, MD: Center for Mental Health Services.

Horvath, A. O., & Bedi, R. P. (2002). The alliance. In J. C. Norcross (Ed.), *Psychotherapy relationships that work: Therapist contributions and responsiveness to patients* (pp. 37–69). New York: Oxford University Press.

Hoyt, M. F. (1978). Secrets in psychotherapy: Theoretical and practical considerations. *International Review of Psychoanalysis, 5,* 231–241.

Hsu, F. L. K. (1981). *American and Chinese: Passage to differences.* Honolulu, HI: University of Hawaii.

Hui, C. H., & Triandis, H. C. (1986). Individualism–collectivism: A study of cross-cultural researchers. *Journal of Cross-Cultural Psychology, 17,* 225–248.

Institute for Mental Health Initiatives. (1995). Family Secrets. *Dialogue: Insights into Human Emotions for Creative Publications, 3,* 1–4.

Jackson, J. M. (1990). The role of implicit communication in therapist self-disclosure. In G. Stricker & M. Fischer (Eds.), *Self-disclosure in the therapeutic relationship* (pp. 93–102). New York: Plenum Press.

Jacobs, T. (1999). On the question of self-disclosure by the analyst: Error or advance in technique? *Psychoanalytic Quarterly, 68,* 159–184.

Johnson, B., Geller, J. D., & Rhodes, R. (1994). Nonverbal profile analysis in psychotherapy: Markers of client-identified misunderstandings. *Psychotherapy, 29,* 54–59.

Johnston, S., & Farber, B. A. (1996). The maintenance of boundaries in psychotherapeutic practice. *Psychotherapy: Theory, Research, Practice, Training, 33,* 391–402.

Jones, E. (1913). The God complex: The belief that one is God, and the resulting character traits. In *Essays in applied psychoanalysis* (Vol. 2, pp. 244–265). London: Hogarth Press, 1951.

Josephs, L. (1990). Self-disclosure in psychotherapy and the psychology of the self. In G. Stricker & M. Fischer (Eds.), *Self-disclosure in psychotherapy* (pp. 75–89). New York: Plenum Press.

Jourard, S. (1964). *The transparent self.* New York: Van Nostrand.

Jourard, S. (1968). *Disclosing man to himself.* New York: Van Nostrand.

Jourard, S. (1971a). *Self-disclosure: An experimental analysis of the transparent self.* New York: Wiley-Interscience.

Jourard, S. M. (1971b). *The transparent self* (rev. ed.). New York: Van Nostrand.

Jourard, S. M., & Lasakow, P. (1958). Some factors in self-disclosure. *Journal of Abnormal and Social Psychology, 56,* 91–98.

Kahn, J. H., Achter, J. A., & Shambaugh, E. J. (2001). Client distress, disclosure, characteristics at intake, and outcome in brief counseling. *Journal of Counseling Psychology, 48,* 203–211.

Kaplan, A. H., & Rothman, D. (1986). The dying psychotherapist. *The American Journal of Psychiatry, 143,* 561–572.

Kazantzakis, N. (1952). *Zorba the Greek.* (C. Wildman, Trans.). New York: Simon & Schuster.

Kelly, A. E. (1998). Clients' secret keeping in outpatient therapy. *Journal of Counseling Psychology, 45,* 50–57.

Kelly, A. E. (2000). Helping construct desirable identities: A self-presentational view of psychotherapy. *Psychological Bulletin, 126,* 474–494.

Kelly, A. E., & Achter, J. A. (1995). Self-concealment and attitudes toward counseling in university students. *Journal of Counseling Psychology, 42*, 40–46.

Kelly, A. E., Kahn, J. H., & Coulter, R. G. (1996). Client self-presentations at intake. *Journal of Counseling Psychology, 43*, 300–309.

Kelly, A. E., & McKillop, K. J. (1996). Consequences of revealing personal secrets. *Psychological Bulletin, 120*, 450–465.

Kempler, B. (1987). The shadow side of self-disclosure. *Journal of Humanistic Psychology, 27*, 109–117.

Khan, M. (1986). Outrageousness, compliance, and authenticity. *Contemporary Psychoanalysis, 22*, 629–652.

Kim, B. S. K., Hill, C. E., Gelso, C. J., Goates, M. K., Asay, P. A., & Harbin, J. M. (2003). Counselor self-disclosure, East Asian American client adherence to Asian cultural values, and counseling process. *Journal of Counseling Psychology, 50*, 324–332.

Knox, S., & Hill, C. E. (2003). Therapist self-disclosure: Research-based suggestions for practitioners. *Journal of Clinical Psychology/In Session, 59*, 529–540.

Knox, S., Hess, S. A., Petersen, D. A., & Hill, C. E. (1997). A qualitative analysis of client perceptions of the effects of helpful therapist self-disclosure in long-term therapy. *Journal of Counseling Psychology, 44*, 274–283.

Kohut, H. (1971). *The analysis of the self: A systematic approach to the psychoanalytic treatment of narcissistic personality disorders.* New York: International Universities Press.

Kohut, H. (1977). *The Restoration of the self.* New York: International Universities Press.

Kowalski, R. (1999). Speaking the unspeakable: Self-disclosure and mental health. In R. Kowalski & M. Leary (Eds.), *The social psychology of emotional and behavioral problems: Interfaces of social and clinical psychology* (pp. 225–247). Washington, DC: American Psychological Association.

Kremer, T. G., & Gesten, E. L. (1998). Confidentiality limits of managed care and clients' willingness to self-disclose. *Professional Psychology: Research and Practice, 29*, 553–558.

Kursh, C. (1971). The benefits of poor communication. *Psychoanalytic Review, 58*, 189–208.

Ladany, N. (2004). Psychotherapy supervision: What lies beneath. *Psychotherapy Research, 14*, 1–19.

Ladany, N., Hill, C. E., Corbett, M. M., & Nutt, E. A. (1996). Nature, extent, and importance of what psychotherapy trainees do not disclose to their supervisors. *Journal of Counseling Psychology, 43*, 10–24.

Ladany, N., & Lehrman-Waterman, D. E. (1999). The content and frequency of supervisor self-disclosures and their relationship to supervisor style and the supervisory working alliance. *Counselor Education and Supervision, 38*, 143–160.

Ladany, N., & Melincoff, D. S. (1999). The nature of counselor supervisor nondisclosure. *Counselor Education and Supervision, 38*, 161–176.

Ladany, N., & Walker, J. A. (2003). Supervisor self-disclosure. *In Session/Journal of Clinical Psychology, 59*, 611–621.

LaFromboise, T., Coleman, H. L. K., & Gerton, J. (1993). Psychological impact of biculturalism: Evidence and theory. *Psychological Bulletin, 114,* 395–412.

Lane, J. S., Farber, B. A., & Geller, J. D. (2001, June). *What therapists do and don't disclose to their patients.* Paper presented at the annual meeting of the Society for Psychotherapy Research, Montevideo, Uruguay.

Lane, R. C., & Hull, J. W. (1990). Self-disclosure and classical psychoanalysis. In G. Stricker & M. Fisher (Eds.), *Self-disclosure in the therapeutic relationship* (pp. 31–46). New York: Plenum Press.

Langs, R. L. (1974). *The technique of psychoanalytic psychotherapy* (Vol. 2). New York: Aronson.

Langs, R. L. (1975). The therapeutic relationship and deviations in technique. *International Journal of Psychoanalytic Psychotherapy, 4,* 106–141.

Langs, R. L. (1978). Validation and the framework of the therapeutic situation. *Contemporary Psychoanalysis, 14,* 98–125.

Langs, R. L. (1984). The framework of training analyses. In R. L. Langs (Ed.), *International Journal of Psychoanalytic Psychotherapy* (Vol. 10, pp. 259–287). New York: Aronson.

Larson, D. G. (1993). *The helper's journey: Working with people facing grief, loss, and life-threatening illness.* Champaign, IL: Research Press.

Larson, D. G., & Chastain, R. L. (1990). Self-concealment: Conceptualization, measurement, and health implications. *Journal of Social and Clinical Psychology, 9,* 439–455.

Leahy, R. L. (2001). *Overcoming resistance in cognitive therapy.* New York: Guilford Press.

Leichtentritt, J., & Schechtman, Z. (1998). Therapist, trainee, and child verbal response modes in child group therapy. *Group Dynamics: Theory, Research, and Practice, 2,* 37–47.

Lepore, S. J., Silver, R. C., Wortman, C. B., & Waymenr, H. A. (1996). Social constraints, intrusive thoughts, and depressive symptoms among bereaved mothers. *Journal of Personality and Social Psychology, 70,* 271–282.

Lethem, J. (2000). *Motherless Brooklyn.* New York: Vintage Books.

LeVine, E., & Franco, J. N. (1981). A reassessment of self-disclosure patterns among Anglo-Americans and Hispanics. *Journal of Counseling Psychology, 28,* 522–524.

Levinson, D. J., Sharaf, M. R., & Gilbert, D. C. (1966). Intraception: Evolution of a concept. In G. J. DiRenzo (Ed.), *Concepts, theory and explanation in the behavioral sciences* (pp. 116–135). New York: Random House.

Lewin, K. (1948). *Resolving social conflicts: Selected papers on group dynamics.* New York: Harper.

Lindner, R. (1955). *The fifty-minute hour: A collection of true psychoanalytic tales.* New York: Bantam Books.

Little, M. (1985). Winnicott working in areas where psychotic anxieties predominate: A personal record. *Free Associations, 3,* 9–42.

Littlefield, R. P. (1974). Self-disclosure among some Negro, White, and Mexican-American adolescents. *Journal of Counseling Psychology, 21,* 133–136.

Livingston, R., & Farber, B. A. (1996). Beginning therapists' responses to client shame. *Psychotherapy, 33,* 601–610.

Lodge, D. (1995). *Therapy: A novel.* New York: Viking.

Loo, C., Tong, B., & True, R. (1989). A bitter bean: Mental health status and attitudes in Chinatown. *Journal of Community Psychology, 17,* 283–296.

Lopez, S. R., & Guarnaccia, P. J. (2000). Cultural psychopathology: Uncovering the social world of mental illness. *Annual Review of Psychology, 51,* 571–598.

Luft, J. (1969). *Of human interaction.* Palo Alto, CA: National Press Books.

Lyall, S. (2005, February 27). Growing up royal: Freud would recognize this family. *The New York Times, Week in Review* (Section 4), p. 2.

Macdonald, J., & Morley, I. (2001). Shame and non-disclosure: A study of the emotional isolation of people referred for psychotherapy. *British Journal of Medical Psychology, 74,* 1–21.

Mahl, G. F. (1977). Body movement, ideation, and verbalization during psychoanalysis. In N. Freedman & S. Grand (Eds.), *Communicative structures and psychic structures* (pp. 291–308). New York: Plenum.

Mann, T. (1936). *Stories of three decades* (H. T. Lowe-Porter, Trans.). New York: Knopf.

Marcus, D. M. (1998). Self-disclosure: The wrong issue. *Psychoanalytic Inquiry, 18,* 566–579.

Markus, H. R., & Kitayama, S. (1991). Culture and self: Implications for cognition, emotion, and motivation. *Psychological Review, 98,* 224–253.

Marmor, J. (1953). The feeling of superiority: An occupational hazard in the practice of psychiatry. *American Journal of Psychiatry, 110,* 370–376.

Marsella, A. J. (1982). Culture and mental health: An Overview. In A. J. Marsella & G. M. White (Eds.), *Cultural conceptions of mental health and therapy* (pp. 359–388). Boston: Reidel.

Mathews, B. (1988). The role of therapist self-disclosure in psychotherapy: A survey of therapists. *American Journal of Psychotherapy, 42,* 521–531.

Mathews, B. (1989). The use of therapist self-disclosure and its potential impact on the therapeutic process. *Journal of Human Behavior and Learning, 6,* 25–29.

McCarthy, P. R., & Betz, N. E. (1978). Differential effects of self-disclosing versus self-involving counselor statements. *Journal of Counseling Psychology, 25,* 251–256.

McCullough, L. V. (1997). *Changing character.* New York: Basic Books.

McCullough, L., Kuhn, N., Andrews, S., Kaplan, A., Wolf, J., & Hurley, C. L. (2003). *Treating affect phobia: A manual for short-term dynamic psychotherapy.* New York: Guilford Press.

McDaniel, S. H., Stiles, W. B., & McGaughey, K. J. (1981). Correlations of male college students' verbal response mode use in psychotherapy with measures of psychological disturbance and psychotherapy outcome. *Journal of Consulting and Clinical Psychology, 49,* 571–582.

McGarty, M. (1988). The analyst's pregnancy. *Contemporary Psychoanalysis, 24,* 684–692.

McGovern, T. F., & Armstrong, D. (1987). Comparison of recovering and non-alcoholic alcoholism counselors: A survey. *Alcoholism Treatment Quarterly, 4,* 43–60.

McNamara, E. (1994). *Breakdown: Sex, suicide, and the Harvard psychiatrist,* New York: Simon & Schuster.

McWilliams, N. (1994). *Psychoanalytic Diagnosis: Understanding personality structure in the clinical process.* New York: Guilford Press.

Messer, S. B. (2002). A psychodynamic perspective on resistance in psychotherapy: Vive la resistance. *Journal of Clinical Psychology, 58,* 157–163.

Messer, S. B., & Winoker, M. (1980). Some limits to the integration of psychoanalytic and behavior therapy. *American Psychologist, 35,* 818–827.

Michener, C. (1995, October 23). They've got a secret. *Time,* p. 98.

Mikulincer, M., & Nachson, O. (1991). Attachment styles and patterns of self-disclosure. *Journal of Personality and Social Psychology, 61,* 321–331.

Miletic, M. (1998). Rethinking self-disclosure. *Psychoanalytic Inquiry, 18,* 580–600.

Miller, H. (1941). Creative death. *The Wisdom of the Heart* (pp. 1–12). New York: New Directions, 1947.

Miranda, J. (1996). Introduction to the special section on recruiting and retaining minorities in psychotherapy research. *Journal of Consulting and Clinical Psychology, 64,* 848–850.

Miranda, J., Azocar, F., Organista, K. C., Munoz, R. F., & Lieberman, A. F. (1996). Recruiting and retaining low-income Latinos in psychotherapy research. *Journal of Consulting and Clinical Psychology, 64,* 868–874.

Mitchell, S. (1995). Interaction in the Kleinian and interpersonal traditions. *Contemporary Psychoanalysis, 31,* 65–91.

Mitchell, S. A. (1993). *Hope and dread in psychoanalysis.* New York: Basic Books.

Mitchell, S. A. (2000). *Relationality: From attachment to intersubjectivity.* Hillsdale, NJ: Analytic Press.

Mitchell, S. A. (2002). *Can love last?: The fate of romance over time.* New York: Norton.

Mitchell, S. A., & Black, M. J. (1995). *Freud and beyond: A history of modern psychoanalytic thought.* New York: Basic Books.

Miyanaga, K. (1991). *The creative edge: Individualism in Japan.* New Brunwick, NJ: Transaction.

Molina, R. A., & Franco, J. N. (1986). Effects of administrator and participant sex and ethnicity on self-disclosure. *Journal of Counseling and Development, 65,* 160–162.

Momigliano, L. N. (1987). A spell in Vienna—but was Freud a Freudian?: An investigation into Freud's technique between 1920 and 1938, based on the published testimony of former analysands. *International Review of Psycho-Analysis, 14,* 373–389.

Moskowitz, S. A., & Rupert, P. A. (1983). Conflictual resolution within the supervisory relationship. *Professional Psychology: Research and Practice, 14,* 632–641.

Muehleman, T., Pickens, B. K., & Robinson, F. (1985). Informing clients about the limits to confidentiality, risks, and their rights: Is self-disclosure inhibited? *Professional Psychology: Research and Practice, 16,* 385–397.

Murphy, K. C., & Strong, S. R. (1972). Some effects of similarity self-disclosure. *Journal of Counseling Psychology, 19,* 121–124.

Murray, B. (2002, June). Writing to heal. *Monitor on Psychology, 33,* 54–55.

Nakanishi, M. (1987). Perceptions of self-disclosure in initial interaction: A Japanese sample. *Human Communication Research, 13,* 167–190.

Newman, C. F., & Strauss, J. L. (2003). When clients are untruthful: Implications for the therapeutic alliance, case conceptualization, and intervention. *Journal of Cognitive Psychotherapy: An International Quarterly, 17,* 241–252.

Nilsson, D. E., Strassberg, D. S., & Bannon, J. (1979). Perceptions of counselor self-disclosure: An analogue study. *Journal of Counseling Psychology, 26,* 399–404.

Noel, R. C., & Smith, S. S. (1996). Self-disclosure of college students to faculty: The influence of ethnicity. *Journal of College Student Development, 37,* 88–94.

Nolen-Hoeksema, S., McBride, A., & Larson, J. (1997). Rumination and psychological distress among bereaved partners. *Journal of Personality and Social Psychology, 72,* 855–862.

Norcross, J. C., & Goldfried, M. R. (1992). *Handbook of psychotherapy integration.* New York: Basic Books.

Norton, R., Feldman, C., & Tafoya, D. (1974). Risk parameters across types of secrets. *Journal of Counseling Psychology, 21,* 450–454.

Oates, J. C. (2001, December 31). Words fail, memory blurs, life wins. *The New York Times,* p. A11.

Orange, D. M., & Stolorow, R. D. (1998). Self-disclosure from the perspective of intersubjectivity theory. *Psychoanalytic Inquiry, 18,* 530–537.

Orlinsky, D., & Howard, K. (1975). *Varieties of psychotherapeutic experience.* New York: Teachers College Press.

Orlinsky, D. E., & Howard, K. I. (1986). Process and outcome in psychotherapy. In S. L. Garfield & A. E. Bergin (Eds.), *Handbook of psychotherapy and behavior change* (3rd ed., pp. 311–381). New York: Wiley.

Ornstein, P. H. (2005). When "Dora" came to see me for a second analysis. *Psychoanalytic Inquiry, 25,* p. 94–114.

Papouchis, N. (1990). Self-disclosure and psychotherapy with children and adolescents. In G. Stricker & M. Fisher (Eds.), *Self-disclosure in the therapeutic relationship* (pp. 157–173). New York: Plenum Press.

Pattee, D., & Farber, B. A. (2004, November). *Gender and client self-disclosure in psychotherapy.* Paper presented at the meeting of the Society for Psychotherapy Research (North American chapter), Springdale, Utah.

Pennebaker, J. W. (1990). *Opening up: The healing powers of confiding in others.* New York: Guilford Press.

Pennebaker, J. W. (Ed.). (1995). *Emotion, disclosure, and health.* Washington DC: American Psychological Association.

Pennebaker, J. W. (1997). Writing about emotional experiences as a therapeutic process. *Psychological Science, 8,* 162–166.

Pennebaker, J. (2002, August). *Expressively easing trauma.* Paper presented at the annual meeting of the American Psychological Association, Chicago.

Percy, W. (1960). *The moviegoer.* New York: Avon.

Plasky, P., & Lorion, R. (1984). Demographic parameters of self-disclosure to psychotherapists and others. *Psychotherapy, 21,* 483–490.

Ponterotto, J. G., Alexander, C. M., & Hinkston, J. A. (1988). Afro-American preferences for counselor characteristics: A replication and extension. *Journal of Counseling Psychology, 35,* 175–182.

Pope, K. S., Sonne, J. L., & Greene, B. (2006). *What therapists don't talk about and why: Understanding taboos that hurt us and our clients.* Washington, DC: American Psychological Association.

Pope, K. S., & Tabachnick, B. G. (1993). Therapists' anger, hate, fear, and sexual feelings: National survey of therapist responses, client characteristics, critical events, formal complaints, and training. *Professional Psychology: Research and Practice, 24,* 142–152.

Pope, K. S., & Tabachnick, B. G. (1994). Therapists as patients: A national survey of psychologists' experiences, problems, and beliefs. *Professional Psychology: Research and Practice, 25,* 247–258.

Pope, K. S., Tabachnick, B. G., & Keith-Spiegel, P. C. (1987). Ethics of practice: Beliefs and behaviors of psychologists as therapists. *American Psychologist, 42,* 993–1006.

Pope, K. S., Tabachnick, B. G., & Keith-Spiegel, P. C. (1988). Good and poor practices in psychotherapy: National survey of beliefs of psychologists. *Professional Psychology: Research and Practice, 19,* 547–552.

Poston, W. S. C., Craine, M., & Atkinson, D. R. (1991). Counselor dissimilarity confrontation, client cultural mistrust, and willingness to self-disclose. *Journal of Multicultural Counseling and Development, 19,* 65–73.

Ramirez, M., III. (1984). Assessing and understanding biculturalism–multiculturalism in Mexican-American adults. In J. L. Martinez & R. H. Mendoza (Eds.), *Chicano psychology* (pp. 77–94). San Diego, CA: Academic Press.

Ramsdell, P. S., & Ramsdell, E. R. (1993). Dual relationships: Client perceptions of the effect of client counselor relationship on the therapeutic process. *Clinical Social Work Journal, 21,* 195–212.

Regan, A. M., & Hill, C. E. (1992). Investigation of what clients and counselors do not say in brief therapy. *Journal of Counseling Psychology, 39,* 168–174.

Reich, W. (1949). *Character analysis.* New York: Orgone Institute Press.

Reik, T. (1948). *Listening with the third ear.* New York: Farrar, Strauss.

Reisner, S. (1991). Reclaiming the metapsychology: Classical revisionism, seduction, and the self in Freudian psychoanalysis. *Psychoanalytic Psychology, 8,* 439–462.

Renik, O. (1995). The ideal of the anonymous analyst and the problem of self-disclosure. *Psychoanalytic Quarterly, 62,* 553–571.

Renik, O. (1999). Playing one's cards face up in the analysis: An approach to the problem of self-disclosure. *Psychoanalytic Quarterly, 68,* 521–539.

Renik, O. (2002, Feb.). *Honesty and dishonesty in the consulting room.* Paper presented at the 13th annual conference of the National Institute for the Psychotherapies, New York.

Rennie, D. (1992). Qualitative analysis of the client's experience in psychotherapy: The unfolding of reflexivity. In S. G. Toukmanian & D. L. Rennie (Eds.), *Psychotherapy process research: Paradigmatic and narrative approaches* (pp. 211–233). Newbury Park, CA: Sage.

Rennie, D. (1994). Clients' deference in psychotherapy. *Journal of Counseling Psychology, 41,* 427–437.

Ridley, C. R. (1984). Clinical treatment of the nondisclosing Black client. *American Psychologist, 39,* 1234–1244.

Robitschek, C. G., & McCarthy, P. R. (1991). Prevalence of counselor self-reference in the therapeutic dyad. *Journal of Counseling and Development, 69,* 469–472.

Roe, D., & Farber, B. A. (2001). Differences in self-disclosure in psychotherapy between American and Israeli patients. *Psychological Reports, 88,* 611–624.

Rogers, C. (1957). The necessary and sufficient conditions of therapeutic personality change. *Journal of Consulting Psychology, 21,* 95–103.

Rogler, L. H., Malgady, R. G., & Rodriguez, O. (1989). *Hispanics and mental health: A framework for research.* Malabar, FL: Krieger.

Roland, A. (1994). Identity, self, and individualism in a multicultural perspective. In E. P. Salett & D. R. Koslow (Eds.), *Race, ethnicity, and self* (pp. 11–23). Washington, DC: National Multicultural Institute.

Rosen, R., & Krotov, M. (2005, April 4). A few things are illuminated: A conversation with literary star Jonathan Safran Foer. *Columbia Daily Spectator,* p. 3.

Rosenblatt, A., & Mayer, J. E. (1975, May). Objectionable supervisory styles: Students' views. *Social Work, 20,* 184–189.

Rosenthal, E. S. (1990). The therapist's pregnancy: Impact on the treatment process. *Clinical Social Work Journal, 18,* 213–226.

Rossner, J. (1983). *August.* Boston: Houghton Mifflin.

Rushdie, S. (1991). *Midnight's children.* New York: Penguin Books.

Russo, R. (1998). *Straight man.* New York: Vintage.

Sabogal, F., Marin, G., Otero-Sabogal, R., Marin, B. V., & Perez-Stable, P. (1987). Hispanic familism and acculturation: What changes and what doesn't. *Hispanic Journal of Behavioral Sciences, 9,* 397–412.

Safire, W. (1999, November 28). On language: Bread 'n' butter. *New York Times Magazine,* pp. 46–48.

Safran, J., & Muran, J. C. (2000). *Negotiating the therapeutic alliance: A relational treatment guide.* New York: Guilford Press.

Safran, J. D., Muran, J. C., Samstag, L. W., & Stevens, C. (2002). Repairing alliance ruptures. In J. C. Norcross (Ed.), *Psychotherapy relationships that work: Therapist contributions and responsiveness to patients* (pp. 235–254). New York: Oxford University Press.

Saltzman, M. (1986). *Iron and silk.* New York: Random House.

Sanders Thompson, V. L., Bazile, A., & Akbar, M. (2004). African Americans' perceptions of psychotherapy and psychotherapists. *Professional Psychology: Research and Practice, 35,* 19–26.

Sandhu, D. S. (1997). Psychocultural profiles of Asian and Pacific Islander Americans: Implications for counseling and psychotherapy. *Journal of Multicultural Counseling and Development, 25,* 7–22.

Saramago, J. (2002). *The Cave* (M. J. Costa, Trans.). New York: Harcourt.

Schore, A. N. (2000). Attachment and regulation of the right brain. *Attachment and Human Development, 2,* 23–47.

Searles, H. (1975). The patient as therapist to his analyst. In P. Giovacchini (Ed.), *Tactics and techniques in psychoanalytic therapy* (Vol. 2, pp. 95–151). New York: Aronson.

Sears, D. O. (1986). College sophomores in the laboratory: Influences of a narrow data base on social psychology's view of human nature. *Journal of Personality and Social Psychology, 51,* 515–530.

Seeley, K. M. (2000). *Cultural psychotherapy.* Northvale, NJ: Aronson.

Seldes, G. (1985). *The great thoughts.* New York: Ballantine Books.

Seligman, M. E. P. (1995). The effectiveness of psychotherapy: The *Consumer Reports* study. *American Psychologist, 50,* 965–974.

Shaffer, P. (1973). *Equus.* New York: Penguin Books.

Shapiro, D. (1999). *Neurotic styles.* New York: Basic Books.

Sharaf, M. R., & Levinson, D. J. (1964). The quest for omnipotence in professional training. *Psychiatry: Journal for the Study of Interpersonal Processes, 27,* 135–149.

Sheese, B. E., Brown, E. L., & Graziano, W. G. (2004). Emotional expression in cyberspace: Searching for moderators of the Pennebaker disclosure effect via e-mail. *Health Psychology, 23,* 457–464.

Shon, S. P., & Ja, D. Y. (1982). Asian families. In M. McGoldrick, J. K. Pearce, & J. Giordano (Eds.), *Ethnicity and family therapy* (pp. 208–228). New York: Guilford Press.

Shonfeld-Ringel, S. (2001). A re-conceptualization of the working alliance in cross-cultural practice with non-Western clients: Integrating relational perspectives and multicultural theories. *Clinical Social Work Journal, 29,* 53–63.

Shostrom, E. L. (Producer). (1965). *Three approaches to psychotherapy (Part 2)* [film]. Orange, CA: Psychological Films.

Silverman, S. (2001). Inevitable disclosure: Countertransference dilemmas and the pregnant lesbian therapist. *Journal of Gay and Lesbian Psychotherapy, 4,* 45–61.

Simi, N. L., & Mahalik, J. R. (1997). Comparison of feminist versus psychoanalytic/dynamic and other therapists on self-disclosure. *Psychology of Women Quarterly, 21,* 465–483.

Simon, J. (1988). Criteria for therapist self-disclosure. *American Journal of Psychotherapy, 42,* 404–415.

Simon, J. C. (1990). Criteria for therapist self-disclosure. In G. Stricker & M. Fisher (Eds.), *Self-disclosure in the therapeutic relationship* (pp. 207–225). New York: Plenum Press.

Simon, R. (1989). Sexual exploitation of patients: How it begins before it happens. *Psychiatric Annals, 19,* 104–107, 111–112.

Simone, D. H., McCarthy, P., & Skay, C. L. (1998). An investigation of client and counselor variables that influence likelihood of counselor self-disclosure. *Journal of Counseling and Development, 76,* 174–182.

Singer, E. (1977). The fiction of analytic anonymity. In K. A. Frank (Ed.), *The human dimension in psychoanalytic practice* (pp. 181–192). New York: Grune & Stratton.

Skolnick, N. J., & Messler Davies, J. (1992). Secrets in clinical work: A relational point of view. In N. J. Skolnick & S. C. Warshaw (Eds.), *Relational perspectives in psychoanalysis* (pp. 217–238). Mahwah, NJ: Analytic Press.

Slavin, R. L. (1993). The significance of here-and-now disclosure in promoting group cohesion in group psychotherapy. *Group, 17,* 143–150.

Sloan, D. M., & Marx, B. P. (2004). A closer examination of the structured written disclosure procedure. *Journal of Consulting and Clinical Psychology, 72,* 165–175.

Smyth, J. M. (1998). Written emotional expression: Effect sizes, outcome types, and moderating variables. *Journal of Consulting and Clinical Psychology, 66,* 174–184.

Snell, W. E., Jr., Miller, R. S., Belk, S. S., Garcia-Falconi, R., & Hernandez-Sanchez, J. E. (1989). Men's and women's emotional disclosures: The impact of disclosure recipient, culture, and the masculine role. *Sex Roles, 21,* 467–486.

Sohn, A., & Farber, B. A. (2003, November). *Patterns of self-disclosure in psycho-therapy and marriage.* Paper presented at the annual meeting of the Society for Psychotherapy Research (North American chapter), Newport, RI.

Spiesman, J. C. (1959). Depth of interpretation and verbal resistance in psychother-apy. *Journal of Consulting Psychology, 23,* 93–99.

Stern, D. (1985). *The interpersonal world of the infant.* New York: Basic Books.

Stiles, W. B. (1984). Client disclosure and psychotherapy session evaluations. *British Journal of Clinical Psychology, 23,* 311–312.

Stiles, W. B. (1987). "I have to talk to somebody": A fever model of disclosure. In V. J. Derlega & J. H. Berg (Eds.), *Self-disclosure: Theory, research, and therapy* (pp. 257–282). New York: Plenum Press.

Stiles, W. B. (1995). Disclosure as a speech act: Is it psychotherapeutic to disclose? In J. W. Pennebaker (Ed.), *Emotion, disclosure, and health* (pp. 71–91). Washington, DC: American Psychological Association.

Stiles, W. B., & Shapiro, D. A. (1994). Disabuse of the drug metaphor: Psychotherapy process outcome correlations. *Journal of Consulting and Clinical Psychology, 62,* 942–948.

Storr, A. (1996). *Feet of clay: The power and charisma of gurus.* New York: Free Press.

Stroebe, M., Stroebe, W., Schut, H., Zech, E., & van den Bout, J. (2002). Does disclosure of emotions facilitate recovery from bereavement? Evidence from two prospective studies. *Journal of Consulting and Clinical Psychology, 70,* 169–178.

Sue, D. W., & Sue, D. (1991). Counseling strategies for Chinese Americans. In C. Lee & B. L. Richardson (Eds.), *Multicultural issues in counseling: New approaches to diversity* (pp. 79–90). Alexandria, VA: American Counseling Association.

Sue, D. W., & Sue, D. (1999). *Counseling the culturally different: Theory and practice* (3rd ed.). New York: Wiley.

Sullivan, H. S. (1953). *The interpersonal theory of psychiatry.* New York: Norton.

Tang, N. (1997). Psychoanalytic psychotherapy with Chinese Americans. In E. Lee (Ed.), *Working with Asian Americans* (pp. 323–341). New York: Guilford Press.

Tangney, J. P. (1990). Assessing individual differences in proneness to shame and guilt. *Personality and Social Psychology, 59,* 102–111.

Tangney, J. P., Wagner, P., Fletcher, C., & Gramazow, R. (1992). Shamed into anger? The relation of shame and guilt to anger and self-reported aggression. *Journal of Personality and Social Psychology, 62,* 669–675.

Taylor, P. J. (1993). Gay men's engagement in psychotherapy as a function of therapist gender and therapist self-disclosure of sexual orientation: An analogue study. *Dissertation Abstracts International, 53*(11-B), 6000.

Taylor, S. E., & Armor, D. A. (1996). Positive illusions and coping with adversity. *Journal of Personality, 64,* 873–898.

Taylor, S. E., & Brown, J. (1988). Illusion and well-being: A social psychological perspective on mental health. *Psychological Bulletin, 103,* 193–210.

Taylor, S. E., Kemeny, M. E., Reed, G. M., Bower, J. E., & Gruenewald, T. L. (2000). Psychological resources, positive illusions, and health. *American Psychologist, 55,* 99–109.

Tennyson, A. (1842). Ulysses. In E. Blunded (Ed.), *Selected poems: Tennyson* (pp. 69–70). New York: Macmillan, 1960.

Terrell, F., & Terrell, S. (1984). Race of counselor, client sex, cultural mistrust level, and premature termination from counseling among Black clients. *Journal of Counseling Psychology, 31*, 371–375.

Thompson, B., & Hill, C. E. (1991). Therapist perceptions of client reactions. *Journal of Counseling and Development, 69*, 261–265.

Thompson, C. (1956). The role of the analyst's personality in therapy. *American Journal of Psychotherapy, 10*, 347–359.

Thompson, C. E., Worthington, R., & Atkinson, D. R. (1994). Counselor content orientation, counselor race, and Black women's cultural mistrust and self-disclosures. *Journal of Counseling Psychology, 41*, 155–161.

Thompson, E. E., Neighbors, H. W., Munday, C., & Jackson, J. S. (1996). Recruitment and retention of African American patients for clinical research: An exploration of response rates in an urban psychiatric hospital. *Journal of Consulting and Clinical Psychology, 64*, 861–867.

Tillman, J. G. (1988). Psychodynamic psychotherapy, religious beliefs, and self-disclosure. *American Journal of Psychotherapy, 52*, 273–286.

Tolstoy, L. (1877). *Anna Karenina*. (Trans. By L. & A. Mande). Franklin Center, PA: The Franklin Library, 1980.

Toukmanian, S. G., & Brouwers, M. C. (1998). Cultural aspects of self-disclosure and psychotherapy. In S. S. Kazarian & D. R. Evans (Eds.), *Cultural clinical psychology: Theory, research, and practice* (pp. 106–124). New York: Oxford University Press.

Triandis, H. C. (1988). Collectivism and individualism: A reconceptualization of a basic concept in cross cultural psychology. In G. K. Verma & C. Bargley (Eds.), *Personality, attitudes, and cognition* (pp. 60–95). London: Macmillan.

Triandis, H. C., Lisansky, J., Marin, G., & Betancourt, H. (1984). *Journal of Personality and Social Psychology, 47*, 1363–1375.

Truax, C. B., & Carkhuff, R. R. (1965). Client and therapist transparency in the psychotherapeutic encounter. *Journal of Counseling Psychology, 12*, 3–9.

Tschuschke, V., & Dies, R. R. (1997). The contribution of feedback to outcome in long-term group psychotherapy. *Group, 21*, 3–15.

Tsujimura, A. (1987). Some characteristics of the Japanese way of communication. In D. L. Kincaid (Ed.), *Communication theory: Eastern and Western perspectives* (pp. 115–126). San Diego, CA: Academic Press.

Tung, M. (1991). Insight oriented psychotherapy and the Chinese patient. *American Journal of Orthopsychiatry, 61*, 186–194.

Turgenev, I. (1861). *Fathers and sons* (R. E. Matlaw, Trans.). New York: Norton, 1966.

Uba, L. (1994). *Asian Americans: Personality patterns, identity, and mental health.* New York: Guilford Press.

Vasquez, M. T. (1994). Latinas. In L. Comas-Diaz & B. Greene (Eds.), *Women of color: Integrating ethnic and gender identities in psychotherapy* (pp. 114–138). New York: Guilford Press.

Vinogradov, S., & Yalom, I. D. (1990). Self-disclosure in group therapy. In G. Stricker & M. Fischer (Eds.), *Self-Disclosure in the therapeutic relationship* (pp. 191–204). New York: Plenum Press.

Vontress, C. E. (1971). Racial differences: Impediments to rapport. *Journal of Counseling Psychology, 18*, 7–13.

Wachtel, P. (1993). *Therapeutic communications: Principles and effective practice.* New York: Guilford Press.

Walen, S., DiGiuseppe, R., & Dryden, W. (1992). *A practitioner's guide to rational-emotive therapy.* New York: Oxford University Press.

Walker, M. M. (1999). Dual traumatization: A sociocultural perspective. In Y. M. Jenkins (Ed.), *Diversity in college settings: Directives for helping professionals* (pp. 51–65). New York: Routledge.

Wallace, E., & Alonzo, A. (1994). Privacy versus disclosure in psychotherapy supervision. In S. E. Greben & R. Ruskin (Eds.), *Clinical perspectives on psychotherapy supervision* (pp. 211–230). Washington, DC: American Psychiatric Press.

Wasserman, M. D. (1999). The impact of psychoanalytic theory and a two-person psychology on the empathizing analyst. *International Journal of Psycho-Analysis, 80*, 449–464.

Watkins, C. E. (1990). The effects of counselor self-disclosure: A research review. *The Counseling Psychologist, 18*, 477–500.

Watkins, C. E., & Schneider, L. J. (1989). Self-involving versus self-disclosing counselor statements during an initial interview. *Journal of Counseling and Development, 67*, 345–349.

Watkins, C. E., & Terrell, F. (1988). Mistrust level and its effects on counseling expectations in Black–White counselor relationships: An analogue study. *Journal of Counseling Psychology, 35*, 194–197.

Wegner, D. M., & Lane, J. D. (1995). From secrecy to psychopathology. In J. W. Pennebaker (Ed.), *Emotion, disclosure, and health* (pp. 25–46). Washington, DC: American Psychological Association.

Weinberg, H. (1988). Illness and the working analyst. *Contemporary Psychoanalysis, 24*, 452–461.

Weiner, M. F. (1983). *Therapist disclosure: The use of self in psychotherapy.* Boston: University Park Press.

Weiner, M. F., & Schuman, D. W. (1984). What patients don't tell their therapists. *Integrative Psychiatry, 2*, 28–32.

Wells, T. L. (1994). Therapist self-disclosure: Its effects on clients and the treatment relationship. *Smith College Studies in Social Work, 65*, 23–41.

Wetzel, C. G., & Wright-Buckley, C. (1988). Reciprocity of self-disclosure: Breakdowns of trust in cross-racial dyads. *Basic and Applied Social Psychology, 9*, 277–288.

Wheelis, A. (1958). *The quest for identity.* New York: Norton.

Wilkenson, S. M., & Gabbard, G. O. (1993). Therapist self-disclosure with borderline patients. *Journal of Psychotherapy Practice and Research, 2*, 282–295.

Winnicott, D. W. (1949). Hate in the counter-transference. *International Journal of Psychoanalysis, 30*, 69–74.

Winnicott, D. W. (1952). Anxiety associated with insecurity. In *Collected papers: Through pediatrics to psycho-analysis.* London: Tavistock, 1958.

Winnicott, D. W. (1960). The theory of the parent–infant relationship. *International Journal of Psycho-Analysis, 41*, 585–595.

Winnicott, D. W. (1965). *The maturational processes and the facilitating environment: Studies in the theory of emotional development.* New York: International Universities Press.

Wise, T. (2004). *Waking up: Climbing through the darkness.* Oxnard, CA: Pathfinder.

Worthington, E. L. (1987). Changes in supervision as counselors and supervisors gain experience: A review. *Professional Psychology: Research and Practice, 18,* 189–208.

Wurmser, L. (1981). *The mask of shame.* Baltimore: Johns Hopkins University Press.

Yalom, I. D. (1970). *The theory and practice of group psychotherapy.* New York: Basic Books.

Yalom, I. D. (1992). *When Nietzsche wept.* New York: Basic Books.

Yalom, I. D. (1989). *Love's executioner and other tales of psychotherapy.* New York: Basic Books.

Yalom, I. D. (1999). *Momma and the meaning of life.* New York: Basic Books.

Yalom, I. D. (2002). *The gift of therapy: An open letter to a new generation of therapists and their patients.* New York: HarperCollins.

Yates, R. (1961). *Revolutionary road.* New York: Vintage Books.

Yeh, C. J., & Hwang, M. Y. (2000). Interdependence in ethnic identity and self: Implications for theory and practice. *Journal of Counseling and Development, 78,* 420–429.

Yerushalmi, H. (1992). On the concealment of the interpersonal reality in the course of supervision. *Psychotherapy, 29,* 438–446.

Yi, K. (1995). Psychoanalytic psychotherapy with Asian clients: Transference and therapeutic considerations. *Psychotherapy, 32,* 308–316.

Yourman, D. B. (2003). Trainee disclosure in psychotherapy supervision: The impact of shame. *In Session/Journal of Clinical Psychology, 59,* 601–609.

Yourman, D. B., & Farber, B. A. (1996). Nondisclosure and distortion in psychotherapy supervision. *Psychotherapy, 33,* 567–575.

Yum, J. O. (1988). The impact of Confucianism on interpersonal relationships and communication patterns in East Asia. *Communications Monographs, 55,* 374–388.

Zeddies, T. J. (2000). Within, outside, and in between the relational unconscious. *Psychoanalytic Psychology, 17,* 467–487.

Zhang, A. Y., Snowden, L. R., & Sue, S. (1998). Differences between Asian and White American's help seeking and utilization patterns in the Los Angeles area. *Journal of Community Psychology, 26,* 317–326.

Author Index

Subject Index